# Miracles on
# Horseferry Road

*For supporting the Anthony
Nolan Foundation and
for my life —
Thank you,
Nancy E. Ternent*

# Miracles on Horseferry Road

## A victory over cancer

## Nancy Ternent

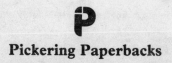

**Pickering Paperbacks**

Copyright © 1985 Nancy Ternent

First published in 1985
by Pickering and Inglis Limited
3 Beggarwood Lane,
Basingstoke, Hants RG23 7LP,
United Kingdom.

*British Library Cataloguing in Publication*

Ternent, Nancy
  Miracles on Horseferry Road: a victory over cancer
  1. Leukaemia—Biography  2. Christian life
  I. Title
  248.8′6    BV4910

ISBN 0 7208 0654 2

Quotations and references used
with kind permission from the Publishers

Phototypeset by Brian Robinson, North Marston, Bucks.

Printed and bound in Great Britain by
Anchor Brendon Ltd, Tiptree, Essex

'For I know the plans I have for you, says the Lord. They are plans for good and not for evil, to give you a future and a hope. In those days when you pray, I will listen. You will find me when you seek me, if you look for me in earnest.'

Jeremiah 29: 11-13
*The Living Bible*

## Dedication

*To my mother, Ian Kirby, Shirley Nolan, Prof. Barratt*
*and my very loving family*
*and with thanksgiving to my Heavenly Father*
*in the hope that all his children*
*may come to know His wonderful love.*

## Acknowledgement

*With gratitude to Peter Jennings*
*for his help and encouragement*

# Foreword

*by Dr John Goldman, Senior Lecturer,*
*Department of Haematology,*
*Royal Postgraduate Medical School, London*

In times of battle some soldiers, not many, are called upon to make decisions that may mean life or death for the troops they command; sometimes these decisions are critical for the soldier's own survival. In peacetime few of us are ever asked to make decisions of any great impact – our problems are usually rather mundane and we are seldom faced with a real choice of life or death. Nancy Ternent in this book has documented the events that led up to just this choice and in doing so she reminds us on almost every page of the precious and uncertain nature of the life we live – in some senses the modern equivalent of the ancient Greek tragedy – but with a happy ending.

Leukaemia is an intriguing disease – it fascinates the professional and captures the imagination of the layman. It is thought to take origin from a single cell in the bone marrow – somewhere in the cavity of the larger bones of the body where blood is normally made. This rogue cell produces many progeny that themselves proliferate and gradually displace all normal blood production. When fully established, billions of these malignant cells fill the marrow spaces and overflow into the blood. Thus leukaemia is easy to diagnose, though frequently unsuspected before the haematologist examines the blood under his microscope. For the professional the fascination lies in the very simplicity of diagnosis and the knowledge that the hidden cause of the leukaemia lies locked in the cell he sees before him, though the key remains elusive. Indeed many scientists believe that discovery of the mechanisms that make a marrow cell leukaemic will lead rapidly to better understanding of the causes of cancer in general.

For the layman the disease fascinates for other reasons. It is rare but strikes without warning. It attacks young children who seem to deserve it least, but it involves adults also. Popularly the diagnosis of leukaemia is seen as a sentence of death. Not all are aware of the major advances made in recent years in the treatment of childhood leukaemia – with genuine cure rates approaching 70%. Fewer still are aware that some adults with leukaemia can also be cured by drug treatment or by bone marrow transplantation, as Nancy's story tells. But one thing is certain. The chance of curing all types of leukaemia will increase in the years ahead and the story told here, unique in its time, may well become tomorrow's commonplace. Let us hope that this is so.

There used to be much debate as to whether a doctor should or should not tell his patient when leukaemia was diagnosed. Such days are past. Without a truthful explanation of diagnosis and treatment plans, only the most skilful of medical manipulators could persuade a patient to accept the rather unpleasant drugs and other manoeuvres necessary to get the leukaemia under control – and then to continue the treatment for many months to achieve total eradication. And to subject a patient to the rigors of marrow transplantation without frank discussion of the alternatives would be unthinkable. In this book Nancy tells the story from the patient's point of view – a viewpoint that doctors do not so much forget as choose sometimes to ignore. The horror of finding that one has leukaemia at a relatively young age; the reactions and responses of family members and friends; the differing approaches of various doctors and the importance of sympathetic nurses; and the very unpleasantness of the treatment and its complications. These are real phenomena which to the doctor seem secondary to the technical aspects of the cure. For the patient they are only too real but the path is undoubtedly smoothed by the professionalism of a specialist unit. No one however can help greatly with the decision of whether one should undergo a highly experimental transplant procedure. At the time when Nancy made her decision, bone marrow transplant was yet more uncertain than it is now. Transplants using family members as donors were often successful but transplants with unrelated donors almost always failed. Yet the alternative seemed even worse. One or two years of disease remission followed by almost inevitable relapse and death. Advice she could seek from many people but the decision Nancy had to make was hers and hers alone.

High technology medicine has advanced greatly in recent years and progress in bone marrow transplantation has been impressive in the last decade. Much of the credit goes justly to Dr Donnall Thomas, working first in Cooperstown in New York and latterly in Seattle. Occasional patients had been treated by transplantation of donor marrow in the 1950s and 1960s but the clinical results were for the most part unconvincing. The sceptics believed that what could undoubtedly be achieved with the experimental animal would never be attainable in man. Dr Thomas, working originally against formidable opposition, treated patients first with aplastic anaemia, a disease of unexplained bone marrow failure, and later patients with leukaemia. Though initially many of his patients died, some survived with evidence that blood production was of donor type. As the years passed it became increasingly clear that aplastic anaemia could be reversed and acute leukaemia could be cured by transplant of marrow from normal donors – though still not in every case. It became clear also that transplant was most likely to be successful when the donor was a brother or sister to the patient – and one who had the same bone marrow type as the patient. In the middle 1970s other groups started very cautiously to follow Dr Thomas's lead. Transplants were performed in Los Angeles, London, Paris and Basel. In these 'early' days, some were successful but many still failed. By 1980 however there were 8 active transplant centres in the USA and 10 or 15 in Europe. Patients transplanted for acute leukaemia were unquestionably being cured and the scene was set for further expansion. In the beginning of 1985 there are at least 10 hospitals in the United Kingdom with the expertise to perform bone marrow transplant for leukaemia or aplastic anaemia; there may be 50 such centres in the rest of Europe and at least a similar number in North America. But many problems remain. Not least is the fact that transplant is still effectively limited to those with matched family members to act as donors. For the professional perhaps the most interesting aspect of Nancy's story is the use of the matched unrelated donor. The optimists hope that this is just a forerunner of routine success not too far ahead.

If transplant is the topic of this book, there is another theme that deserves mention. Nancy has learned some spiritual lessons. Her strength to take the decisions she made and the courage she needed to continue at times when prospects looked grim came in large part from her conviction that God was her supporter. The doctors who plan the strategy of treating leukaemia and transplanting bone marrow sometimes come to believe that they influence events more than they really can. What doctor knows who will get leukaemia? What doctor knows which of his patients will survive a transplant, and which die? Or why?

London, January 1985

# Part One

'So I then told him how, one day, I met a young ant called Claudia, who was limping. We were in the garden at home. With her permission, I turned her over on her back to see what was the matter with her tiny foot.

'So it was that Claudia for the first time saw the sky – for ants are just like us – go, go, go, run, run, run, never pausing to look up and gaze at the sky!

'On seeing the sky for the first time, Claudia lay open-mouthed with amazement and delight. I soon realized there was no point in asking her about her foot. She wasn't listening. She was looking at the sky.'

Dom Helder Camara
*A Thousand Reasons for Living*
(Darton, Longman & Todd, London, 1981)

# 1

The word seemed to be coming toward me through a cloud: hazy, indistinct, blurred around the edges. Who had said it? What did it mean? Not wanting to hear, I pleaded, 'Please say it again.'

Through this mist I saw my husband George standing beside my bed, felt his hand warm, holding mine. Then I heard his voice, quiet, dry, without inflection, 'The doctor says you have leukaemia.'

Then, as he held me close in his arms, the meaning of the words began to penetrate my mind. I have leukaemia? Is it me he's talking about? Me? No, George was wrong. It was Daddy who had leukaemia, not me. Sometimes I dreamed of him. This must be a dream.

I sank back onto the pillow. The clouds enfolded me and I drifted away.

*     *     *     *

'Jesus loves me, this I know,' crooned my toy Donald Duck in a squeaky voice. He sat with Theodore, my teddy bear, a scruffy toy cat, my doll Luvums and me in a cosy circle presided over by my mother. I was four and I had a cold so we were having Sunday School at home.

The year was 1944 and that Sunday was cold and rainy in Omaha, standing where the Oregon Trail crossed the Missouri River at the edge of the prairieland which gently

13

rolled across Nebraska to the foothills of the Rocky Mountains. Most of the land was now given to growing corn and cattle and Omaha's stockyards were second only to Chicago's. In those days Mother considered it safe to send me by trolley bus at the age of five all the way to my Daddy Bill's printing shop. Daddy Bill was my grandfather and his shop was in a rather poor area of the city, a haunt of cowboys no longer with ranges to ride. Mother cautioned me against speaking to strangers, but I used to chat amiably with the cheerful tramps sitting along the wall where the trolleys stopped, sipping something from brown paper bags. I was a bit frightened, though, of the Indians one could still sometimes see wrapped in blankets and with feathers in their felt hats – standing aloof and gazing far away as if they could still see the open ranges.

On other Sundays, without any regularity, I was taken to the Sunday School at the Presbyterian church. I remember memorizing the twenty-third Psalm, but it puzzled me that we should pray to a shepherd we did not want.

Grace was said only at the special feasts for which the whole family gathered together to celebrate Thanksgiving, Christmas and Easter. It was always the 'task' of one of the children to bless the food. Intuitively I knew that it embarrassed the adults to pray aloud. Maybe prayer, and, it followed, religion itself, was just something for children like Santa Claus and the Easter Bunny, but without the gaiety. Perhaps it was a solemn and uncomfortable duty.

Heaven, on the other hand, ranked in my imagination with the Land of Oz, a happy, magical place. You got there by faith. There was an invisible staircase that led right from my garden up in the air to heaven. You had to look up all the time you were climbing it and just believe that the stairs were there under your feet or you would fall back to the earth. I was very disappointed when Mother told me Daddy Bill wouldn't be able to take his beloved old Ford to heaven with him. I prayed that when it was my turn to climb the stairs God would let me bring Theodore. Otherwise, I wasn't sure I wanted to go.

When I was ten my parents and I (and Theodore) moved to New York city. There I became aware that there were other religions. I had two close girlfriends, we were an inseparable trio, one a Roman Catholic, the other a Jew. It seemed to me that they enjoyed a lot of religious holidays which exempted them from attendance at school. And they had special rules and special foods which set them apart. There wasn't anything special about being a Protestant. In fact, it was rather dull.

It was while we were living in New York that I had my first glimpse of heaven. It was in a dream. We couldn't have a dog, of course, in our apartment in New York, and more than anything in the world that's what I wanted. I prayed for a dog every night. In my dream I went to heaven to ask God for one. There was a shiny tiled walk around a clear, still, pool and Moses was sitting beside it. At one end of the pool was a palace with an open porch and on the porch was a big throne. I sensed, rather than saw, a presence on this throne. But I saw sitting beside the throne a small red spaniel. Then the dream dissolved.

Two years later we moved back to Nebraska, first to a small town called Mead. My parents told me that I could have a dog now. In fact, Mother had found a little dog who had not been treated well by some neighbours who wanted to be rid of it and she hoped I would like it. It was a little red cocker spaniel called Ginger.

The church in Mead was Lutheran and we didn't go very often. The altar of the church was dominated by a life-size statue of Christ painted in natural colours, bright red blood painted around the holes in his hands and feet where the nails had been. It really captured my adolescent imagination. When I was twelve I went away for a week to their summer Bible Camp. I was so inspired by what I learned there that I came home full of zeal and the desire to become a missionary in Africa. My worried family quietly discouraged this and eventually the flame was extinguished.

Once we had settled back in Omaha, both my parents and I became regular attenders of the Methodist church. I was then fourteen and by the time I was fifteen, I had rebelled against Christianity as I then understood it.

In Sunday School classes until then I had always been among the most inquisitive. Sometimes I asked questions which the teachers could not answer as I tried to work out the real meanings of Biblical passages and teachings., I soon realized that much of the Bible was written in symbolism and its interpretation was an exercise in which my mind delighted.

At the Methodist Sunday School the teenagers held their own services and took it in turns to give the sermon. When my turn came, I spoke on my own theory of Genesis and Evolution. After church I was told by an elderly and much-respected gentleman who taught at the Sunday School that his class was very impressed with my presentation and that it had taken him the entire class period to convince them how wrong I was. Now I can see that the incident was simply his mishandling of a sensitive teenager, but at the time it seemed to me that there was no freedom of thought in the church and I stopped attending.

More importantly, though, by this time I could not bring myself to recite the Apostle's Creed or accept the doctrine of the Trinity. Deuteronomy 6:4 says, 'Hear, O Israel: The Lord our God is one Lord.' It seemed to me to be a betrayal of God Himself to pray to anyone else, even Jesus. My search for a religion that would bring me into close communion with God alone had begun.

That same summer I went with my parents to Estes Park in the Rocky Mountains of Colorado where Daddy was attending a conference on industrial psychology. One of the speakers was Aaron Levenstein, a very distinguished Jewish psychologist. He and Daddy became friends and he often spent his evenings in our cabin in conversation dominated by psychology and philosophy. He included me in these conversations, listening to me and speaking to me as though I were an adult. It was flattering and made me feel special, particularly when he gave me a book, far above me intellectually, and which I still treasure today for his inscription, 'To Nancy – who is growing toward the light as all life should'.

But his very goodness itself brought me more doubts and questions concerning God and how to worship Him. My thoughts were very confused as I left our cabin one day and walked up into the mountains to get away and think by myself.

Aaron Levenstein was a good man, but he was a Jew. Did that mean that he wouldn't get to heaven? Was there a heaven? Or a hell? It seemed selfish that people should only be good and do good things for others in order to obtain a heavenly reward or to avoid divine punishment. Could God condemn Aaron Levenstein to hell only because he was not a Christian? What about all the people since time began and in foreign countries who had never heard of Jesus? Could the God I was supposed to love condemn them? I couldn't. How could He? As I climbed up the mountain my mind turned these things round and round, patternless and disconnected like dry leaves swirling in the wind.

Exhausted, I threw myself face-down on a big boulder and wept my despair. I wanted so much to know God, to love Him. But would I ever know who He was and what He wanted? As if in answer, the warm rock beneath me seemed to be breathing and alive, and I felt myself to be in the Father's embrace. A wonderful sense of peace washed over me and I just *knew*: the earth is the living body of God and

17

He loves and will care for all of His creatures, from the tiniest insect to each of His people. We belonged to Him. It was not for me to know *how* He would care for each of us, but I knew now that He would, with love and compassion.

Knowing He was real intensified my quest for a religion I could follow whole-heartedly. Ramakrishna, a Hindu philosopher, said, 'As one can ascend to the top of a house by means of a ladder or a bamboo or a staircase or a rope, so diverse are the ways and means to approach God, and every religion in the world shows one of these ways. Different creeds are but different paths to reach the Almighty . . .' Through books, I set about exploring them all.

In my sixteenth summer, one night as I lay awake in bed, I had a vision. In front of my open eyes I could see a glowing, yet brilliant, light in the darkness that embodied a figure I somehow knew was Jesus. There were no audible words, but a 'voice' spoke to me saying, 'Without me, you will die. If you close your eyes and lose me, you will die.' It was spoken softly and without menace, but I tried to stay awake, to keep my eyes open. Finally, sleep overcame me. Of course, I did not die. I woke up and everything was outwardly just the same. After a few days the vague feeling of uneasiness evaporated and the whole experience was consciously forgotten, pushed aside by other things more real and important: my studies, boyfriends, dances and parties and, ultimately, my twin loves of drama and travel.

But my search for God continued. Along with Theodore and one of Mother's special meatball sandwiches, I carried it with me when I went away to the University of Nebraska in 1958. Besides my majors in English and Drama, I took courses in philosophy and comparative religion. I was inspired by Hesse's *Siddhartha*, bewildered by D. H. Lawrence's *The Man Who Died*, enthralled by the Jewish philosopher Spinoza, touched by the sacrifice of Albert Schweitzer and attracted to Hinduism through the study of the Upanisads, the Vedanta and the Bhagavad-Gita. All contained aspects of the unity which I was seeking.

I wasn't sombre or reclusive. I was attractive, popular and completely involved in the social life on the campus. But sometimes, when the Catholic chapel was empty, I would go in alone to think or pray. Holding the feet of a statue of sweet St. Francis of Assisi, I would long for a way to make sense of all I was learning. And though I found excuses to avoid attending church services with the other members of my sorority, I was elated when, only because of my popularity and seniority, they elected me as their Chaplain. I opened the first meeting with a prayer to Ahura Mazda from the Zoroastrian religion! But always my source of guidance was the Old Testament which I never doubted to be the true, if not the only, word of God.

After graduation in 1962, I spent six months at my parents' new home in Miami, pursuing my acting career and saving money from my clerical job for my first travel adventure. With parental misgivings, at the age of twenty-two I set out alone on the Greyhound bus taking three months to zig-zag north and south across the United States from Miami to San Francisco. Although I settled in San Francisco at the height of the Hippy movement, I was too naïve and childlike myself to relate to these alien 'Flower Children'. And, I was in love . . .

David was Jewish, a twenty-six year-old law student. Though we found more interesting things to do and talk about than religion, I did learn a lot about Judaism from him and found I wanted to know more. When I was lucky enough to land a job with the U.S. Army Special Services and get posted abroad, I decided to try an experiment. Since no one at the base in Germany to which I was assigned knew me, I would pretend to be Jewish and see what it was really like.

Almost at once I sensed a 'differentness' in the way

people regarded me. Especially, being in Germany heightened my awareness of what it meant to be a Jew. I felt a strong sense of identification through my sympathy with the Jews as I toured the concentration camps with their mass graves, furnaces and photographs of atrocities. I studied the religion with deep sincerity and found that I could accept it wholly. In both their sufferings and their triumphs, their practices and beliefs, I felt at one with the Jews. At the end of the year, on my return to San Francisco, I made a formal conversion at the temple and took Rachel as my Jewish name. My family were sorely disappointed, but always remained loving.

When I went to Bangkok as a teacher in 1967, I regarded myself as totally Jewish and was an accepted part of the small Jewish community there. I was even a Sunday School teacher. Since no teaching is permitted on the Sabbath (Saturday), religious instruction is given on Sunday. At home I did not keep strictly kosher but I followed most of the traditions: a mezzuzah on the door, lighting the Sabbath candles, observing customs of the holidays and the meaningful celebrations of life and abstaining from eating pork and shellfish. I felt at home and at peace with no barriers between myself and God. And though I never thought of Jesus as the Messiah, my knowledge of Judaism illuminated His life and teachings. I even tried to incorporate some of His teachings into the way I practised Judaism.

Through living in Bangkok and travelling widely in the Far East, I was among Buddhists, Christians, Hindus and Moslems, but their religions no longer had any appeal for me except as quaint practices and ideological curiosities. Mother, who had by now become a born-again Christian, was fearful that I would be influenced by these 'heathen walking in darkness'. And all her entreaties to me to come back to Jesus fell on deaf ears. I was a Jew.

I met George in Tokyo, and before I married him in 1974 I asked him if he believed in God. He said he did and though he was only nominally a Christian, the answer seemed good enough to someone as much in love with him as I was. To accommodate our differences in beliefs, I composed the wedding ceremony myself. On a warm Florida day standing under magnificent live oaks festooned with Spanish moss beside a small lake, we were joined by a Justice of the Peace.

George was in the British Army. Travelling with him, homemaking and having two babies and being married to a person who didn't practise any religion led to my gradually dropping my Jewish observances. I began to turn to the Bible only in moments of imagined or trivial crisis. Without realizing it, I was drifting further and further away from God. But, praise the Lord, *He* never let go of *me*!

# 2

Travelling with George from posting to posting in the Army was an exciting way of life. In three years we had moved from London to Northern Ireland to Nepal to Belgium.

While we were in Nepal in 1976, our son Cameron was born. The small cantonment in the foothills of the Himalayas with its lovely warm climate, fresh, fresh air – and servants to do the housework! – was the perfect place for a first-time mother, particularly at my age. I was thirty-six. It was ideal for the baby, too. I hated leaving when we were posted on to Belgium in 1977, but it did bring me a few thousand miles closer to my parents. They came to visit us at our Army quarters near Antwerp and to celebrate Cameron's first birthday in October.

Still in Belgium, our second child was due in July 1979. This time my parents intended to be with us when the baby was born. I was thrilled at the prospect because being an only child I knew how disappointing it had been for them to have me always so far away.

In April, though, I had a letter from Mother saying that they would not be able to come after all as Daddy had commitments at work which were unavoidable. By this time, Daddy had also become a born-again Christian and she assured me that they were both praying for me and *knew* that God would give me a safe and easy delivery.

In fact, it was frightening, painful and a near miss.

At the end of June I was admitted to the closest British Military Hospital, the RAF Hospital at Wegberg, Germany. The baby had stopped growing and I was told that labour would have to be induced. The first attempt at this went wrong and, after seven hours of painful labour with no results, was stopped. A week later they said they would try again. As it was near the date, I asked the doctor if he could arrange to do it on July 12th, my father's birthday, thinking what a special gift it would be for him. My parents were in Omaha just now, I thought, visiting the family.

George and Cameron came to the hospital on the day, armed with brown paper bags of sandwiches to await the great event. George wanted to witness the birth as he had done with Cameron's. But after eight hours of labour, the baby had not moved and its heartbeat was becoming alarmingly slow and faint. I was so frightened for the baby, crying as I kissed Cameron and George goodbye as they wheeled me off for an emergency Caesarean. I was prepared to give up my own life if it meant saving the baby.

During the operation it was discovered that the umbilical cord was wrapped around the baby's neck three times. It was a tiny baby girl. Had she been born normally, the cord would have strangled her.

Before she had been properly 'cleaned up' they wheeled her from the theatre to the nursery. Cam, disappointed already that she was a girl, watched her go past and complained to George, 'She's all rusty!'

It was certainly not a 'safe and easy delivery'. But I had to admit that it surely was a miracle. When the hospital chaplain held a 'thanksgiving service' for the newborn babies and their mothers, I could not restrain my tears of gratitude to God for bringing us both safely through it.

George sent a very happy birthday telegram to Daddy and Mother and they replied with their own telegram of excited congratulations.

Before Kirsty was three weeks old, I had another telegram, this time from Mother alone. Without further explanation it said, 'If you want to see Daddy at his best, the doctor says to come in the next two weeks.'

I was so worried as my fearful imagination began to slot the pieces of the puzzle together. My parents couldn't come to Belgium, but they had gone to Omaha. A doctor? See Daddy at his best? I knew what to expect when after two days I was finally able to get through to Mother on the telephone. Daddy must be seriously ill.

But I wasn't prepared when she told me he had leukaemia.

I hung up the phone in a state of shock. I didn't know anything about leukaemia except that children got it and it was nearly always fatal. I looked it up in my friend's encyclopaedia but the entry was brief and confusing. Only one word stood out from the page: 'fatal'.

Kirsty still hadn't received a birth certificate from the German authorities, but within seventy-two hours the British Army had her fully documented and had put me and the two children on the first flight available from Brussels to London. From there, we travelled to Brize Norton Air Force Base by train, where we were put on an indulgence flight to Washington D.C. We had to spend the night there and flew on to Omaha the next morning. Upset at that delay, I was even more disappointed when I could not see Daddy immediately upon my arrival. Mother told me that the doctor had advised Daddy to rest that day so that he could come home for a few hours the following day.

I think Daddy didn't want me and the children to see him in hospital. And, in retrospect, the extra time gave me a chance to talk to Mother and better prepare myself for our meeting.

'Home' was at my Aunt Lillian's and Uncle Benny's where the children and I would be staying. Mother was sleeping on a camp bed in Daddy's private hospital room in order to spend as much time as possible with him and to help in his care.

It was a beautiful Sunday, very hot as summer days in Nebraska are. I wasn't sure what to expect as I waited for Daddy, but apart from being a bit thinner and having lost a little of his hair, he was the same handsome man I had known all my life. He chatted and smiled, even teased, and seemed to really enjoy the lovely dinner Lillian had prepared, though he didn't eat a lot, I noticed.

Naturally he was delighted to see Cameron again and he fell in love with his 'birthday baby girl'.

After dinner Daddy lay down to rest. In a little while I followed him into the bedroom and sat beside the bed. The curtains were drawn against the hot August sun and the room was dim and cool with the air-conditioning on.

I hardly knew what to say or what to talk about. My heart was full of pity and fear and love that could not form itself into words. I wanted us to drop our roles of father and daughter so that we could talk as friends. Yet, as his daughter, I wanted to ask his forgiveness for having spent so much of my life abroad and away from him. Indirectly, we touched upon this and I felt the release of his forgiveness and understanding. And so much love it hurt.

That was the last time that Daddy and I were alone together and so much had been left unsaid. I now found myself a not altogether willing member of an unspoken 'pact' made by the family that Daddy must not be allowed to know how serious his condition was. At the same time, I felt sure that he did know but wanted to spare us his own doubts and fears. Somehow we all managed to pretend to each other that this wasn't really happening, that soon Daddy would get well and everything would be just as before. I never had the courage to break this silent agreement though there was so much I wanted to ask him about and to share with him in the short time we had.

During the weeks I spent in Omaha I grew close to my family once more. The years of our separation dissolved as we shared our lives and hopes again. In seeing familiar homes, streets, buildings, faces, my childhood came alive once more and I had a renewed sense of identity and belonging.

All the family gave wholeheartedly of their time and attention to see to all our needs – caring for us, loving us and praying for us without ceasing.

My cousin Janet took over most of our domestic needs, making her home our home. She was always there with cheerful understanding and consolation and hot food when I returned from the hospital each day. Along with Aunt Lillian and Uncle Benny, Aunt Betty and Uncle Roger were my chief baby-minders and chauffeurs for my daily visits to the hospital. Great-aunt Daisy in her eighties prayed for us constantly. Above all, my cousins JoAnne and Diane gave Daddy their blood, along with strangers I could never know or thank.

JoAnne's was not just a simple donation of whole blood. It required her being on a leukopherhesis machine for two or more hours at a time while blood was taken from a vein in one arm, run through the machine to separate off the particular cells Daddy needed and then returned through a vein in her other arm. I was full of admiration for her for being able to go through this ordeal so willingly. Though I dreaded doing this myself, I had the same blood type as Daddy and pleaded with the doctors to be allowed to do this. They refused me as it was too soon after the Caesarean. I wanted so much to do something for Daddy and I felt so helpless. Holding Kirsty in my arms, I longed to hold and comfort Daddy. And Mother. It was her courage and unwavering faith in Jesus that held all of us together.

How did she and Daddy pass all those long hours alone in

his hospital room? I was sure that they read the Bible and prayed together. I knew that they watched the Lawrence Welk show and must have reminisced about the days when Daddy was a musician and Mother sang with his dance band. Childhood sweethearts, they had known and loved each other for nearly fifty years. But did they ever talk about the possibility of death – just between themselves? Through all those days of hope for a healing, of despair over chemotherapy that didn't work, blood tests and trans-fusions, other tests, X-Rays, infections – short steps forward and longer steps backward, Mother never lost hope. All of us were worried about her. We wanted her to be able to cry and release the awful tension under which she was keeping up such a brave front. It was her unwavering faith that maintained her and us.

I longed for that same kind of faith. I participated in the family's prayer meetings and never stopped praying alone for Daddy's healing. I prayed with the evangelical minister who came to visit Daddy. Finally, I even went to a service at his church. At the end of the service I knelt at the altar rail and cried. I wanted so much to believe in Jesus so that Daddy could be healed. I prayed to God and promised Him that if He would heal Daddy I would become a Christian. Later that day I told Daddy what I had done.

He smiled at me in gentle amusement. 'You can't make bargains with God,' he said.

Even after five weeks I was reluctant to leave, but George's father had died unexpectedly and Daddy told me that I must go to be with George and comfort him.

How precious the love of my family. The night before I left Aunt Lillian baked me my favourite banana cream pie. I didn't know that it would be the last gesture of love that I would receive from her – here.

# 3

I went back to Belgium in September. Mother and Daddy stayed on another month in Omaha, but Daddy was never able to get a remission and the doctors had nothing else to try. In October they went back to Florida and Mother continued to care for Daddy at home. Though I had to rely on a friend's telephone, I talked to Mother as often as possible. Daddy had suffered often from terrible chills and fevers, and I felt badly that in my circumstances there was no way I could be of more use than to try to comfort Mother. There never seemed to be an occasion for me to talk to Daddy himself as she always told me he was resting. As the months wore on, sometimes now there were tears in Mother's voice. Her facade of optimism was beginning to crumble, yet her faith seemed to be increasing. It was hard for me to understand.

When I telephoned in early January 1980, there was no answer. Instinctively I knew that something was wrong. I tried Aunt Lillian in Omaha but she couldn't give me any information. Finally the Belgian operator was able to get through to the hospital in Tallahassee and Daddy himself answered the telephone.

I wish I could remember that conversation. It was very brief and I do remember him assuring me that he was all right. The only actual words I remember were when we tearfully said goodbye and Daddy said, 'I love you for calling'.

Just two days later, Mother saw him through the door of his hospital room. His arms were outstretched and he was speaking rapidly as though to someone he could see, but too quietly for Mother to be able to distinguish any words as she went in to him. A few hours later, he died.

In a dream about that time I saw Daddy sitting under a tree throwing a ball for Ginger. He looked about twenty-five and was smiling. Ginger, who was twelve when she died, gambolled like a young puppy.

There was no comfort in my grief. No solace in my mourning. Only my children brought me brief moments of sunshine, momentarily piercing through the clouds of depression which enveloped me.

I felt personal guilt for Daddy's death. When I had prayed with my family and other Christians in Omaha they had stressed that whatever was asked in the name of Jesus would be given – *if* the person praying had faith that it would really come to pass. I did not have that faith when I prayed for Daddy. I had let him down. My lack of faith, I felt sure, had prevented his healing.

I couldn't understand either why God would let my lack of faith be a consideration in saving Daddy from death. Nor how all this could have happened to a man who loved the Lord as much as my father did.

In every theatre there is a 'green room' where cast, crew and director meet after the curtain is down to discuss the evening's performance – what went well, what did or didn't work and why. Perhaps heaven will be a sort of green room where we can meet after this performance in 'life'. Perhaps there we can discuss it all, find out the Playwright's intentions and how well we fulfilled them, be given explanations and a chance to ask for forgiveness and understanding from Him and from those we have known while here on earth. I hope that this is so.

*

In April we were posted to Aldershot where George worked in the Pay Office of the Cambridge Military Hospital, or the CMH.

By the time Mother came to visit us in July, I had reconciled myself to Daddy's death and been able to rationalize and submerge my feelings of doubt and guilt. Mother and I confined ourselves to recalling the good times.

Mother was still with us when my name came up on the list and I went into the CMH for a routine sterilization. It was August, the month of my fortieth birthday and I didn't want to risk having any more children. I was glad to have Mother there to look after Cameron and Kirsty for the two or three days I might be in hospital, probably even less time if things went well.

But they didn't.

The day before the laparotomy, only a minor operation, a routine blood test was given. A few hours later I was told that the laboratory had detected a slight abnormality in my blood and instead of the operation, Major Winnick would do a bone marrow aspiration the following morning. That same afternoon I also became aware of a soreness in my groin and thought maybe I had strained a muscle.

When Mother visited me that evening I told her only that the operation had been postponed for a day or two as I had a slight fever with a cold coming on. Now I understood the family's pretences during Daddy's illness. How could I frighten Mother by mentioning blood tests and bone marrow?

That next morning I fainted. I put it down to nerves brought on by remembering descriptions of Daddy's bone marrow tests and by my own fear of needles. The idea of having a needle inserted into my breastbone to extract some marrow sounded particularly horrifying. To my relief, I was slightly sedated and it wasn't nearly as ghastly or painful as I had anticipated.

By the afternoon, though, it was quite clear that I was very ill with a high fever caused by an abcess forming in my groin. Mother reluctantly returned home on schedule and I was placed in isolation until the abcess became operable.

I was in isolation for a total of five weeks before and after the operation. My blood was tested daily and I soon lost my fear of, though not my distaste for, needles.

I didn't know how closely God was watching over me already. Had I had the laparotomy on schedule, the incision might have passed through the abcess and could have resulted in peritonitis possibly causing death.

Of course, all the blood tests revived my old misgivings about Daddy's death. Like newly watered flowers they sprang up to accuse me. It was my white blood cells that were abnormal and I feared the worst, but the blood tests showed that I definitely did not have leukaemia. I cried with relief. For I had begun thinking that maybe my strong feelings of guilt could cause me to punish myself by getting leukaemia. Feelings like these can never be explained rationally, nevertheless they seem very logical to the person experiencing them.

I was so relieved at not having leukaemia that I didn't even mind celebrating my birthday in hospital though it certainly wasn't what I planned. Like every other woman I rather dreaded turning forty and I had decided months before that I would meet middle age head-on. I had been dieting and planned to change my hairstyle and revamp my wardrobe. I would get out of the house and do some volunteer work, pursue a stimulating hobby and, of course, be the perfect wife, mother and housekeeper.

That's the way I visualized it. Instead, I was sitting up in a hospital bed with a small sterilized cake from the hospital kitchens. I could only see George's eyes above the mask he was required to wear along with the gown, cap and boots as I was still in isolation. And I could only see the children

31

through the glass windows that lined one wall of my room.

Before I went home in mid-September feeling perfectly fine, I heard Kirsty say her first real words through the glass, 'Bye-bye'.

# Part Two

'EMILY: Good-bye, Good-bye world. Good-bye, Grover's Corners . . . Mama and Papa. Good-bye to clocks ticking . . . and Mama's sunflowers. And food and coffee. And new-ironed dresses and hot baths . . . and sleeping and waking up. Oh, earth, you're too wonderful for anybody to realize you. Do any human beings ever realize life while they live it? – every, every minute?
STAGE MANAGER: No. The saints and poets, maybe – they do some.'

Thornton Wilder
*Our Town*
Longman Group Limited, London, 1977

# 4

The second of November 1980 was a cold, grey Sunday. It was the day before the presidential election in the United States and it made me feel vaguely homesick though it had been fifteen years since I had left America to live and travel in Europe and the Far East. Such a long way I had come on my travels, I mused, as shivering I gathered in the laundry. I did not know that on this day I was embarking on another journey of a different sort.

It felt as cold inside our Army quarter in Aldershot as it was outside, though I seemed to be the only one to think so. I had on a woollen pullover but soon added a cardigan. As the hours passed, I heated another cardigan over the gas fire and put that on as well, but I still felt very, very cold.

At four o'clock I went out into the even colder kitchen to prepare dinner. As I bent over the oven to put in the chicken, I suddenly felt weak and dizzy. I asked George if he minded keeping an eye on the chicken for me while I went upstairs to lie down for a little while before dinner. I crawled under the covers with all my clothes on, thinking only of keeping warm. I didn't wake to finish preparing dinner. I didn't even wake to eat it . . .

I was wakened by George, surprised to find that it was Monday morning. I still had on all my clothes of the day before and now I felt horribly hot with an aching pain in the area of my left shoulder blade. Still, I told George that if he would take three-year-old Cameron to playschool on his way to work, I could pick him up at lunchtime. I was sure that I would be able to manage looking after sixteen-month-old Kirsty.

The next thing I remember was kindly Dr. Watson from the Army Families Medical Clinic standing over the bed. It was already lunchtime, but I had no recollection of how the morning had passed. My eyes focused on Dr. Watson's friendly, weathered face and familiar tweed jacket. He had his worn leather medical bag with him, but still I wondered why he was here. I told him I was feeling much better. But when I tried to sit up so that he could examine me the pain in my shoulder blade and chest was unbearable and my head swam to the point of nausea. Dr. Watson shook his head as he read the thermometer. Immediately he called an ambulance.

Now it was night time and I had staggered out of a bed on Ward Nine at the CMH. I remember a nurse reassuring me that everything was all right as she tucked me back in bed. When I opened my eyes again, the room was full of machinery and I was lying on a table, not a bed. I had been transferred to Intensive Care.

Wires were attached to my chest and I was fascinated watching my heartbeat on a television monitor, oblivious to why this was being done. I felt faintly amused when Major Winfield tested my awareness by asking me such silly questions. 'What was my husband's name? Had I any children?' Why was I having so much difficulty answering him? The words I was trying to say were not the words I heard coming out of my mouth. Major Winfield asked me how old I was. I struggled to answer him and finally I said, 'A hundred years'. What I meant was that I felt ageless, as if I had always existed and always would.

As I drifted in and out of consciousness, there seemed to be two of me. One of me was in my body, ill and in pain.

The other me was standing behind and above my body watching everything with interest. Needles for intravenous drips startled both Nancys into intensely painful oneness from time to time. Horrible bouts of chills, too, brought on awareness. I found it interesting that I was wrapped in the same sort of aluminium material used by astronauts. Though I couldn't eat, I was told that I kept asking for a special American kind of chicken noodle soup. When it was finally located and prepared one of the nurses told me I had only two spoons of it, said it was lovely and drifted away again.

Meanwhile the doctors were kept very busy in trying to make a diagnosis. It had already been established that I had double pneumonia but for a while they were in the dark as to why I seemed unable to fight it. I had been in Intensive Care for seven days when Major Winfield called in Major Gravett of the Haematology Department at the Queen Elizabeth Military Hospital in Woolwich to confirm his diagnosis of acute myeloid leukaemia.

Sirens. Another ambulance. George and a nurse were with me. I was curious to find an oxygen mask over my face, but it was only a fleeting response. George smiled at me. He said we were going to London. I liked London.

But London was a small, green room. A room in Westminster Hospital just off Horseferry Road. George was there but I wondered what had become of the children. George told me that Cameron and Kirsty were all right and that Mother was coming to see me. I told him that it was silly to bother her as I would be better soon and anyway we were going to America for Christmas. We already had the reservations. I don't remember what George answered, but I do remember that it was soon after that that he told me I had leukaemia.

Suddenly, there Mother was! Standing in my room, still wearing her hat and coat. I wondered how she had arrived so quickly. It seemed only minutes ago that George had told me she was coming.

What must Mother have suffered on that long flight alone across the Atlantic? In January she had lost Daddy to leukaemia. In June she was nursing her only sister, my dear Aunt Lillian when she died of a severe stroke. Now her only child had leukaemia as well and was close to death. Was she reliving those terrible memories? Had she come to be with me for the same reason I had gone to be with Daddy? Was I dying?

I left the hospital room and went walking in a wood. The sky was coldly grey and a chilling wind caused the dry, brown leaves to swirl around my feet. I was walking down a long tunnel formed by bare naked branches of almost leafless trees interlaced over a well-trodden earthen path bordered by withered grasses and weeds. The only colours, brown and grey, spoke of death and desolation.

At the end of the tunnel a heavy wooden door, arched and with an iron grill in it, stood partially open. I approached it and put my hand against the rough wood.

Beyond the open doorway I could see only an empty landscape, unbearably sad – the ground sparsely covered with dead grass, a few stunted and bare trees, the sky now nearly white with cold, the mournful wind finding nothing to stir.

I was about to push the door open and go inside when it swiftly banged shut in my face. I fled from the reverberating noise of the slamming door, racing backward up the tunnel and found myself safely back in bed.

This was not a vision or another dream. It was a very real experience. I knew that through that door lay death and that what I had glimpsed on the other side of it was hell. Not fire and torment, but a complete cutting off from God. I knew that if I had gone through that door I would have been damned, dead in both body and spirit, never to know communion with God.

I was frightened. I had denied Jesus many more times and more seriously than had the apostle Peter. I had sinned without recognizing it as sin and with no thought of repentence. With stunning clarity I knew that I had not been saved!

As soon as Mother came to visit me again, I interrupted her greetings and urgently told her that I wanted to be saved. Holding my hands tightly in her own she fervently prayed with me. With tears of gratitude, I accepted God's forgiveness for my sins and asked Jesus to come into my life. At once, I felt His perfect peace.

# 5

Being at Westminster Hospital was further evidence of God's loving care.

Because he had been working closely with Dr. A. J. Barrett, Major Gravett was able to put me under his care immediately. Dr. Barrett is one of the world's leading figures in the treatment of leukaemia and I was truly blessed to be a patient of his and his team of doctors in haematology. Together they formed an international cast: Dr. Mahendra Desai from Bombay, Dr. Ozai Halil from Istanbul, Dr. Rajeev Joshi from Simla and Dr. Jim Kendra from Portsmouth, all places I had been in my travels. Dr. Barrett himself is from London.

My condition, though I did not know it at the time, was described as 'moribund', that is 'in a state of dying'. I was being 'fed' and kept alive entirely intravenously. George and Mother agreed wholeheartedly with the doctors that they should try anything that might restore me.

The pneumonia had entirely blocked my left lung. Someone held me upright while the lung was punctured from the back to drain off the fluid. Was it nature's protection that cushioned the intense pain? Or the Lord's?

Remembering how little Daddy was told, I asked the doctors to be completely honest with me about my treatment and what to expect from it. I begged them not to try to spare my feelings by withholding anything from me and they complied with my wishes. In this way, I felt that I had some control over my body and its treatment and could participate in fighting against my illness. Some of the facts were pretty grim, but I feel it is a violation of the patient's rights concerning himself to treat him with anything other than complete honesty. One wants time to prepare for death; time to say goodbye.

Dr. Barrett decided to risk a course of chemotherapy. It might kill me or I might come through it. If I did get through it, there was just a chance that I might get a remission from the leukaemia. I was dying anyway so there was nothing to lose.

Mother had fastened a small gold cross on a chain around my neck. Inside my gown was pinned a handkerchief that had been anointed with oil as a proxy for me by the elders of her church. Not good luck charms, but visible reminders of the salvation that was already mine. Mother told me to hold fast to Psalm 116:

*'I love the Lord because he hears my prayers and answers them. Because He bends down and listens, I will pray as long as I breathe . . .'*

The chemotherapy was very rough, causing nausea, fevers and chills.

*'. . . Death stared me in the face — I was frightened and sad . . .'*

The course of chemotherapy lasted ten days. I marked them off with brightly-coloured numbers four-year-old Cameron made for me. Each day one number was put up on the wall where I could see it and it reminded me that I really must get well to care for my children. I hoped that making the numbers for me would help Cameron to understand that I hadn't abandoned him.

Finally the ten days were over. I was still alive. We awaited the results.

At last a morning came when all five doctors crowded around my bed. I wouldn't have been surprised if they had burst into song, so joyful was their mood as they repeated over and over to each other and to me, 'It's a miracle!'

I was in remission.

After they left, I cried as I read again the lyrics of Psalm 116:

> '. . . How kind He is! How good he is! So merciful, this God of ours! The Lord protects the simple and the childlike; I was facing death and then He saved me. Now I can relax. For the Lord has done this wonderful miracle for me. He has saved me from death, my eyes from tears, my feet from stumbling. I shall live! Yes, in His presence – here on earth!'

Soon after I was brought into remission, the pneumonia completely disappeared. There followed long days of continual I.V. drips of medication and nutrients. I had been on I.V. since being admitted to Intensive Care at the CMH. The chemotherapy was also administered by I.V. My veins were collapsing one by one and re-siting the needles was becoming increasingly painful. While the needles were being changed I concentrated all my attention on a poster Mother had put on my wall. It pictured a little duckling peeking out of a blue denim shirt pocket and said, 'Lord, protect me and keep me close to your heart'.

I was still running a fairly high temperature which delayed my having a follow-up course of consolidation chemotherapy. I daydreamed about lying on a beach with the warm, yet refreshing, sea lapping over my body. It had a soporific effect on me and brought back cherished memories of other beaches I had known in the South Seas. I imagined I was scuba diving again, dipping under the cool water to follow the fishes. In this way, I tried to will my temperature down.

After several days my temperature did begin to come down. Though I had to stay on the drip for medication and fluids, it was marvellous when I felt hungry again and could begin to eat a little. When everyone was trying to encourage my appetite, I was asked what would taste especially good and I said grape juice. In America this is quite a common drink, but in England in 1980 it was not so easy to come by. Undaunted, Mother finally found some at a religious supply house that stocked it for churches preferring a non-alcoholic communion wine.

When my temperature had at last remained normal for a few days, I was ready for the consolidation therapy. This was to be a five-day course of chemotherapy to ensure the results of the first course which had led to my remission.

A houseman warned me that the drug *daunorubicin* which would be used for the consolidation therapy could make me feel quite nauseous and that I probably wouldn't feel like eating. So the night before it was due to begin I had a little feast of Ritz crackers and grape juice and stayed up late watching a film on the television in my room. I wanted to make myself tired hoping that I could sleep through as much of the anticipated discomfort as possible. After the first day's therapy, though, I felt all right and when George came in on the second day with a take-away hamburger for his lunch, *I* ate it.

At last all my veins gave out and I had to have the last few doses of therapy by sub-cutaneous injection which was a very painful ordeal. Words often quoted by Aunt Lillian: 'He never gives us more than we can bear,' helped me through this and many other dreadful experiences.

Being transfused with blood platelets brought on uncontrollable teeth-shattering chills until this was

43

corrected with prior injections of puriton and hydro-cortisone. Another drug reaction caused a horrible itchy rash all over my body so that I felt on fire and could only escape in snatched moments of dozing.

Finally free of the intravenous apparatus, I was encouraged to get out of bed and walk about in my room. At first I could only walk around the bed, hanging on to it for support as my muscles got used to holding me upright again. I caught a glimpse of myself in the mirror over the wash basin. It was a shocking sight. I wondered how anybody had been able to look at me and smile.

Shakily, I began to start using a little lipstick and eye shadow each day. They only emphasized my skeletal features. Still, this effort encouraged the doctors as it was a positive indication of my will to recover. They even allowed a nurse to wash my hair, and they told me I should be able to go home for Christmas.

As I got stronger I worked on a Christmas stocking I was making for Kirsty to go with the one I had made for Cameron. I was overjoyed at the thought of being able to see them hung up at home. On December 19th, George and Cameron came in a taxi to take me home.

After nearly seven weeks in isolation, the noise of the traffic and the speed of the taxi overwhelmed me. The antibiotics I had been given made my ears ring and the shrill little voices of the children made me wince. But how wonderful to hold them again, to walk through my own front door and see the Christmas tree and Mother and Kirsty waiting with a lovely hot lunch.

I didn't have much appetite and found everything very tiring. Wrapping a few Christmas gifts and playing with the children exhausted me. I slept every afternoon.

We always have our big dinner on Christmas Eve. I couldn't eat much, but enjoyed every morsel I did have, especially the pumpkin pie with whipped cream, the traditional American Christmas dessert that Mother made specially. I was pleased to see that Cameron liked it, too.

Christmas day was beautiful: up at dawn with the children to see what Santa Claus had brought, filled stockings hanging from the mantle, toys and gifts under the tree. Since George had done all the Christmas shopping, I was as happily surprised as they were. All my own presents seemed to be nighties, slippers and dressing gowns. Even a V-shaped pillow for sitting up in bed. That was from George, along with a box of lacy lingerie that really lifted my morale.

The day passed joyfully and, too quickly, it seemed, the children were tucked into their beds. I was looking forward to watching the Morcambe and Wise Special on television but was having a great deal of trouble staying awake. That made me suspect I might have a temperature and I was right. It was 104 degrees. George called the CMH and an ambulance was sent for me.

My holiday was over, but I had had the best of Christmas no matter what the New Year might bring.

# 6

Major Winfield met me at the Cambridge Military Hospital on Christmas night. I felt terribly sorry about spoiling his holiday when he had been so kind to me in November. Back I went to the same room on Ward Nine where I had first been admitted with pneumonia nearly eight weeks ago. Paradoxically, it seemed like years ago in terms of experience, but only minutes ago in its familiarity. Familiar, too, were the needles and the intravenous drips which were begun again.

On New Year's Eve, George got permission to come back to the hospital to see me just before midnight. He knew that celebrating the coming in of the New Year had always been important to me and it was a wonderful surprise to have him there, his arms around me as we listened to *Auld Lang Syne* playing on the radio, and we kissed as far-off church bells proclaimed the beginning of 1981. I had no idea what this New Year would bring. I was only grateful that I was still here to find out.

I continued running a fairly high temperature and was treated with both pills and I.V. for a 'non-specific' infection. I was also given transfusions of whole blood and transfusions of platelets. That was followed by a course of anti-biotic injections, two injections each day for sixteen days. After all that, it was decided that there was no real infection and that my fever had been caused by the strength of the drugs used for the consolidation therapy. It was dying cells that had raised my body temperature. The team at Westminster Hospital had expected some reaction of this sort, but nothing so severe. Now that they knew, they would cut down the strength of the drugs when I began maintenance therapy. That would be a monthly three-day course of chemotherapy and was to begin in February.

Mother had planned to leave right after Christmas but stayed on when I went back into hospital. It was wonderful to have her with us, helping George to look after the children and encouraging me. At the end of every visit she prayed with me, reinforcing my new faith. I was still one of St. Paul's 'baby' Christians, (I Cor. 3:1).

Working downstairs in the CMH Pay Office, George could pop in to see me from time to time during the morning. He worked through the two-hour lunch break and then went home for the day. Mother spent every afternoon with me and George came again in the evening.

Even so, I had many hours alone in which to consider the important decision now facing me. That was whether or not to have a bone marrow transplant, if indeed that were possible.

Dr Barrett is a pioneer in the relatively new field of bone marrow transplantation. The possibility of my having one had been mentioned to me before I left Westminster Hospital in December, Dr. Kendra stating that it offered my only chance of 'real' survival. It sounded dreadful and I hadn't even wanted to think about it. Later, though, I asked Dr. Desai what would happen if I didn't have a transplant. He was truthful, yet reassuring, as he told me that on a programme of maintenance therapy I might stay in remission for as long as two years and that a few people had stayed in remission even longer. However, the remission might only last six months or less. A second remission would be more difficult to attain. A third remission would be almost impossible.

At my insistence, Dr. Desai continued. If I failed to respond to chemotherapy, death was inevitable. They would try to make me as comfortable as possible and lessen the pain with drugs but they could do nothing else; cold and hard facts only softened by his gentle and quiet voice.

In mid-January, just before I was released from the CMH, I went with George and a nurse to the Westminster Hospital for a meeting to discuss my future treatment and the possibility of my having a bone marrow transplant. George didn't see the necessity of his coming, but I wanted him with me. Naturally, Mother was curious to know what was said. As she had to stay at home with the children, I made a tape recording of the conference.

It was a cold day, the sky dark with rain. The Haematology Department on the windowless lower ground floor of the hospital made a gloomy setting, the waiting room walls a muddy shade of beige, its gaudy orange chairs containing ghosts of bald-headed people in drab winter clothing. It all added to my sense of dread. I knew chemotherapy would cause me to lose my hair too, but would I become as lifeless as they seemed to be? I felt the stares of their haunted eyes on my back as we passed them to walk down the narrow corridor to the door of Dr. Barrett's office.

Our meeting was with Dr. Kendra and Major Gravett. Dr. Kendra did most of the talking and the conference lasted for nearly two hours.

Unlike a transplant of a distinct organ such as a kidney or a heart, a bone marrow transplant is a lengthy procedure which does not involve major surgery. Dr. Kendra's descriptions were chillingly realistic as he outlined this procedure day by day. Because I asked for complete truth, he covered every detail including what could go wrong, what might produce adverse reactions and in what ways they would affect me.

The first problem would be to find a suitable bone marrow donor for me. Whenever possible it was a close relative, usually a brother or a sister. I didn't have either and Mother was ruled out as she had had cancer of the breast. They would have to look for an unrelated donor, as near a perfect match as possible. A half-matched donor could cause a particularly disastrous death. Since the facilities for doing bone marrow transplants are, unfortunately, very limited, people with suitable related donors have priority. However, if a donor could be found I would be added to their waiting list.

The testing for an unrelated donor is extremely meticulous and requires a great deal of time. At that time the Anthony Nolan Foundation had a register of about 37,000 willing donors. My blood could be tested against the blood of ten potential donors at a time. As my blood was a fairly common type, Dr. Kendra felt the chances of finding a suitable donor were fairly good.

Assuming that a donor was found, on the first day after being admitted I would be given a test dose of radiation. The following day I would be taken to the operating theatre and have a Hickman's catheter inserted through my neck into my superior vena cava, the large vein which leads directly to the heart. Through this long tube medication could be administered and blood samples extracted, thus eliminating all needles. I found the prospect of a tube in my neck particularly abhorrent. Dr. Kendra told me that, in fact, they caused no pain and that in the Children's Ward the kids went around twirling them like watchchains. That description didn't make me feel much better. Under the anaesthetic I would also be given a lumbar puncture which might cause me to come around with a severe headache, and another bone marrow aspiration. By now I had had several of these.

The next day I would rest and on the fourth day the

immune suppression treatment would commence. This would consist of large doses of very strong chemotherapy over a period of two days. Because it was likely to make me quite ill, I would be mildly sedated and plenty of fluid would be given along with the drugs necessitating the more usual sort of catheter.

Another day of rest and on the seventh day I would be taken to the Royal Marsden Hospital for Total Body Irradiation. A normally lethal dose of radiation would be given to me over a period of seven or eight hours so that it would not kill me, though it, too, would make me feel quite sick. A few hours later on the same day I would be given the donor's bone marrow by intravenous transfusion.

'By magic,' Dr. Kendra said, 'the bone marrow from the donor transfused into the bloodstream finds its own way to the marrow of the recipient's bones'. If the graft is successful it will start to reproduce and destroy any remnants of the diseased bone marrow that may have escaped the killing effects of the chemotherapy and radiation. It will then begin producing healthy new blood cells.

The first few weeks following all this would be a time of wait and see while I would be kept in isolation until all the blood counts proved to be good and the new immune system began taking over the body's protection.

The greatest danger of a bone marrow transplant is *Graft vs. Host* disease. With an organ transplant, the body may reject the new heart or kidney. With a bone marrow transplant the reverse might happen. In Dr. Kendra's words, the lymphocytes from the donor may start screaming that they are in the wrong place. If this happened they would not only reject my system but also attack and destroy it as they would any foreign body. The milder effect of *Graft vs. Host* disease is usually itchy red skin that could start peeling off both internally and externally. Internally it mainly affects the membranes of the gut and liver causing diarrhoea, vomiting and severe abdominal pain.

Dr. Barrett was just then one of the few doctors being allowed to test a new drug called Cyclosporin A, a drug that would lessen the chances of getting *Graft vs. Host* disease. I was told that I could expect to take this oily, unpleasant tasting drug orally twice a day for one hundred to one hundred and fifty days.

Among the side effects of the transplant, my hair would definitely fall out but would grow again in four or five months. I would go into an early menopause which would be dealt with by hormone replacement therapy and I would become sterile due to the radiation. There was a possibility that I might develop cataracts of the eye and that my lungs might be affected by the radiation. The doctors had no way of knowing the longer-term effects because as yet no one had survived long enough to assess them.

Dr. Kendra told me that of the transplants done with unrelated donors and without Cyclosporin A, four had died. When I asked how many had lived, he told me none. They had only done four. But, he explained, that besides not having Cyclosporin, they had all had other problems as well. They had done sixteen transplants on patients with related donors who had the same type of leukaemia as I had and fourteen of them had survived the transplant procedure itself for varying lengths of time. Most had other problems which contributed to their death. I would be the first one to have a transplant in an initial remission which should increase the odds of its success.

Finally, there was no guarantee that even after a successful transplant the leukaemia would not come back.

Today, many types of leukaemia can be treated, controlled or even cured by tablets alone, but that was not so in my case. My only alternative to a transplant would be Maintenance Chemotherapy.

Dr. Kendra explained that chemotherapy was improving every day but that in my case it could never be seen as a cure or even a long-term solution. And it would adversely alter the 'quality' of my life.

This was the message that came across by the time the conference was over: If a donor could be found, go for a transplant; if not, don't give up hope as chemotherapy was improving all the time.

While the doctors were talking, I had done my best to be brave. But sometimes quiet tears had escaped my eyes as I visualized all these things happening to me. Going back to the Cambridge Military Hospital, I felt only numb and detached, as if it had been someone else we had been talking about.

For awhile, I couldn't even think about it. What a good thing it was that I had made a tape of the conference for Mother. I didn't have the courage to listen to it for some days, but when I did I was able to comprehend all the information and to see it more objectively. I still found it very frightening though.

In my 'mind's eye' the narrow white corridor leading to the door of Dr. Barrett's office became another tunnel. Standing by the door the doctors were beckoning me to enter, Dr. Kendra with his bushy beard looming large in the front. Behind me the corridor was sealed off. There was no escape and I felt heart-pounding panic.

Still at the CMH, I questioned everyone and considered carefully all the advice I was given. Some doctors were against the transplant but most of them favoured it. It never bothered me to talk openly with friends or staff at the hospital about the probability of my death. I knew from my wonderful experience that I now had nothing to fear in death itself.

Stated simply, if I had a transplant I had a fifty-fifty chance between the leukaemia being cured or a relatively quick death. On Maintenance Therapy my life might last a little longer but death was inevitable and would be uncomfortably prolonged. Ultimately, I knew the decision could only be mine, but deciding between these alternatives was far from simple.

Maybe the Lord had healed me while I was in Westminster Hospital. Certainly it had seemed so. My current blood tests showed no indication of leukaemia. The doctors were sure I had it and told me so, but there was no way they could prove it to me. Had I *really* had leukaemia or had I only *seemed* to have it, a self-inflicted punishment for my lingering feelings of guilt over my supposed part in causing Daddy's death? If I really had had leukaemia, and if Jesus had truly healed me, a transplant would not only be an unnecessary and senseless risk, it would show yet again my lack of faith. These feelings I couldn't discuss with anyone. Even to me they sounded somewhat irrational.

I just didn't know what to believe. I didn't have the courage to stop my treatment and see if I still had leukaemia. I prayed. I decided to trust the doctors and that if a donor were found it would be a sign from God that I did need a transplant.

On January 17th 1981 I was well enough to go home. Again, I prayed. I telephoned the Westminster Hospital and told them I had decided to have a bone marrow transplant.

# 7

On January 22nd Mother flew back to the States and I reported to Westminster's Haematology Department and gave my first blood sample to be used in their search for a suitable donor for me.

Britain is the only country in the world which has a register of potential bone marrow donors. This is entirely due to the courage, persistence and love of Mrs. Shirley Nolan and the support given to her by Dr. David James. In December 1971 her son Anthony was born with Wiskott-Aldridge Syndrome, a rare bone marrow disease for which there was no cure. Though her baby was given no chance to survive, with the devoted love and care of his mother, he went on living. In 1973 a remarkable medical breakthrough was made at Westminster Children's Hospital in London. Professor Humble had administered a bone marrow transplant on a little boy with a condition similar to Anthony's. The little boy was Simon Bostic and at that time the transplant was thought to be a success. On hearing about it, Shirley Nolan flew with Anthony from Australia to London to give her son his only possible chance to live. She did everything in her power to find a compatible donor for Anthony and the story is movingly told in her book *A Kiss Through Glass* (Mirror Books 1979). For six years she searched in vain for a donor, but Anthony had a rare blood tissue type and tragically he died just before his eighth birthday. So selfless is her love that she continues still her work for the benefit of others. She established the Anthony Nolan Laboratories with its register of bone marrow donors in the grounds of St. Mary Abbot's Hospital Kensington to which she and Dr. James and his wife give all of their time even today.

Again, I felt it was a special blessing that I was here in England, close to the Anthony Nolan Laboratories and under the care of Westminster. Of all the places in the world where I had been, this was the best possible place I could be now.

My Maintenance Therapy was rescheduled and the following day, January 23rd, I went back to the CMH for my first course. This time I could walk the short distance up the hill from home.

I was to have one dose of intravenous chemotherapy each day for three days, each dose taking about two hours. I could have gone home at the end of each day's treatment, but as I still didn't feel very strong I decided to stay in the hospital for the entire three days.

The only pain it caused was in finding new sites for the needle as the veins in my arms were now of no use. The needle was usually put in one of my hands using a very small needle and a 'giving set' of the type used for babies. This time the drugs made me nauseous and caused vomiting. They also made me very tired and a little irritable and weepy so I was glad that I had decided to stay at the hospital. It would have been unfair to subject George and the children to all this.

Every four weeks then, I would check into the Cambridge Military Hospital after George had come home at lunchtime on Friday, and I would return home on Sunday evening. George and the children came up for a short visit on Saturday mornings. If I was unable to have a bone marrow transplant, this is the routine I would continue to follow until I had a relapse. I tried not to think about that.

I used these quiet weekends in hospital to rest, to read the Bible and refresh myself spiritually and to write letters in a place where I could concentrate more easily than at home. I wrote letters to all of my family in the 'States and to all of my friends scattered around the world. Briefly I told them what was happening to me. I tried to tell them how I really felt about them, how much they meant to me and how much I loved them. I wrote about the good times I had shared with each of them and told them emphatically that although I was fairly optimistic about the transplant, I was not afraid to die and why.

George said, 'After writing all those things to everybody, won't you feel a bit silly if you survive?' I did laugh with him, but if I did survive what would feeling a bit embarrassed matter anyway? Ordinarily we take each other so much for granted. It's good to take the time to tell people how really appreciated they are. I was glad that I knew what was going to happen and thankful that I had the time to write these letters.

Still, I could not avoid thinking during these long hours on my own. I understood now what Dr. Kendra meant about the 'quality of life'. 'Maintenance' therapy: to keep me in the same state. How long could I endure it? How long would it last? Would I be able to get a second remission? a third?

My thoughts were never suicidal, but many times I felt that if my life was going to end it would be better if it ended now, before my children grew to love and need me any more. Now they were young enough to forget me quite easily, though that realization hurt, and with two appealing little children George was still young enough to find someone else. I even fantasized that he might marry my single cousin, Janet. She would make a marvellous mother for my children! Most of all, though, dying now would save my husband and my family the heartbreak and emotional strain of a prolonged illness. And it would save me also from the unknown suffering that must lie ahead.

I tried to leave those thoughts behind me at the hospital each time I finished a course of therapy and walked back down the hill on a Sunday evening. At home between times I determinedly picked up the routines of my normal life – if it could still be called that.

It took a long time to get my energy back. At first just getting dressed in the morning took me nearly an hour and left me in need of a rest before I could begin attending to Kirsty. George took Cameron to playschool on his way to work in the morning and brought him home again at lunchtime. For the first month we had a home help for a few hours each week, but found it easier to manage ourselves. I did the light housework and George helped out with the heavier chores on the weekends.

With the possibility of so little time left the feeling that I should do something 'significant' with my life began to gnaw at me. It had always been my desire to do something for the benefit of humanity in general. But what I might do had always seemed vague and far-off. With sudden panic I realized that my 'someday' was *now*! Now was the only time I had left, and I still didn't know what I could do. There wasn't time to write a great novel or paint a masterpiece even if I had the talent, which emphatically I did not. I had no money with which to endow my favourite charities and no opportunities for accomplishing any worthwhile public service. Throughout my very enjoyable life I had done so many of the things that I had wanted to do – I had no regrets of that kind. But what had I ever done for others? And what could I hope to do now?

Then I came across these words of Helen Keller on duty: 'I long to accomplish a great and noble task, but it is my chief duty to accomplish small tasks as if they were great and noble'. And so I set myself to my own small tasks and began to find the fulfillment that had eluded me for so long.

Though I tried always to appear cheerful, I had my down days, of course. But early on I realized that self-pity was a waste of time and a terrible imposition on others. I was going to make whatever time I had left enjoyable for myself and my family and friends.

Most of the time I was surprised at how easy this was. Each day I saw anew just how much I had to enjoy. Pushing a pram full of giggling Kirsty every morning as I began taking Cameron to his playschool myself became a new source of pleasure, even though it was uphill all the way. And the harder it became for me, the more joy I found in it. Coming down the hill after school I would give them both a freewheeling ride in the pram, all of us laughing at every bump. And so it was with all my routine tasks because *I* was there and *I* was doing them. Paradoxically, because I had less time I had more time, for important things.

It was spring. I planted flowers in our garden. With hitherto uncharacteristic patience, I encouraged the children to help me. If I went away, I hoped the flowers would remind them of these happy days. If I came home I could visualize myself convalescing in the sunny flower-filled garden.

These thoughts about my illness coloured all I did, quite naturally, but they could not dominate my will to enjoy life. I planted more flowers.

I'll be the first to admit that I really let the housework slide. Not that I ever let anything get really dirty, but the house did acquire a nice, cluttered lived-in atmosphere. I had got my priorities straight at last. I sat in the sunshine and watched my children playing while the house more-or-less kept itself.

I even enjoyed making out a new will. Instead of lumping together all my worldly goods, I carefully considered each item and left it to the person I thought would like it best. In this way, too, I revisited my past and all the places I had been.

Maybe it was selfish or egotistical, but I wanted each of my children to have something to remember me by. I had begun making Cameron a patchwork and embroidered quilt cover while I was in isolation at the Cambridge during the last summer. I set myself the goal of finishing it working very late each evening until it was complete.

Cameron accidentally broke one of my favourite possessions. I wasn't angry with him. Possessions were no longer important. Holding the pieces of the figurine in my hand, I felt only a deep sadness. My life was fragile, too. Maybe I would be broken like this little angel. As if they had been spoken aloud, I heard the words, 'This is my body which is broken for you,' and I felt peace. Jesus would be holding me in His hand, just as I held this figure. As a mother holds and tenderly nurses a sick child, so Jesus holds each of us gently in His arms and soothes us. Not only does He give us comfort but He gives us the strength to fight and the will to live. We don't have to ask. He is always there, waiting for us to turn to Him, to climb upon His lap as a little child. I mended the angel. I knew Jesus would mend me. And I told Cameron this, wiping away his tears as he watched me.

Though we try to ignore it, we all face physical death from the moment we are born. However, when illness brings us face to face with it, it is not easy to take it as a matter of certainty unless it is put into perspective in the light of living for eternity. Then it has its compensations in a heightened awareness of all the good things that are already ours and of all the possibilities there are to explore as we school ourselves for all that is yet to come after we have finished our temporal lives. It is much harder on family and friends because they must strive to appear

59

optimistic, wearing a mask of hope, even maintaining a sense of humour for the benefit of a loved one who is ill, no matter what they themselves know or fear. Just as in wartime, fighting against a common enemy can bring people closer together. But George and I seemed to be growing further apart.

God provided me with just the sort of friend I needed when a new neighbour, Anna Bishop, called on me one day in early March. When she learned that I had leukaemia and what my prospects were, she accepted my illness in the same matter-of-fact way that I had, and it never interfered with the quality of our friendship. Together we played with our children and shared the duties of looking after them. We shopped together and had long discussions over coffee. Like me, Anna was struggling toward an acceptance of Christianity. With her I felt safe to discuss the few remaining doubts I still had as my intellect tried to grasp the reality of the miracles I had already received.

In my heart I knew these miracles were valid, but Satan was trying to convince me that they were my own imagination. Sometimes I could feel a deathly presence hovering over my shoulder. When I whirled around to confront it, it had always vanished. I wanted to scream with rage – but at what? At cancer? At Satan? I couldn't see my enemy. But if my enemy was in my mind, Jesus was still in my heart.

Anna's growing faith strengthened my own. Together we planted more flowers.

For Kirsty I began a tapestry to commemorate her birth. I spent many pleasant hours working on it out-of-doors while she played or sat beside me dreaming in the grass. I dreamt of my own childhood and wondered what Kirsty dreamt of. She tangled up all my tapestry wool and we both laughed at the colourful mess.

Having been a conscientious calorie counter most of my

life, imagine my delight when Dr. Kendra told me that if I were lucky enough to get to have a transplant I should put on an extra twenty pounds or so so that I could afford to lose as I probably would during the transplant procedure. What bliss to eat as much spaghetti and ice cream as I liked. Cam and I made pizzas so loaded with goodies they could only be eaten with spoons!

A visit to the dentist in April cut short my new pleasure in eating. I had been strongly advised by my doctors to have my teeth thoroughly checked and attended to prior to the possible transplant. I couldn't help the tears sliding down my cheeks as the dentist explained to me that I had areas of exposed bone that were a high infection risk so that I would have to have *nine* of my back teeth taken out. It wasn't a suggestion, it was imperative. My heart sank. I had already lost almost all of my head of long hair and now I was going to lose all these teeth. It made no difference that the dentist said that the smile I could not muster now would not be diminished by their loss. It was as if 'it' was taking little bits of myself — not just my blood, my hair, my teeth, but chipping away at the very cement straining to hold me together.

When I got home from the dentist George told me that Major Gravett had called and said that Westminster thought they might have found a near-perfect donor.

I couldn't plant more flowers. It was snowing.

I pasted warm memories into long-neglected scrapbooks. The snow went away and it was warm again. I took the children for a picnic.

It was only a paper bag lunch of peanut butter and jam sandwiches, crisps, apples and fruit juice and we only went to the little park quite close to our quarter. But Cam was as excited as if we were in another world. And as we all played on the swings and sat in the grass to eat, we *were* in another world alone and quite apart. It gave me the most wonderful feeling when Cameron said to me, 'We're enjoying ourselves aren't we, Nancy?' For a moment I felt more like his best friend than his mother, a moment I will always cherish.

Very early in the year I had scoured the local library for books about cancer. They were interesting until I remembered why I was reading them. The only one that mentioned bone marrow transplants described this treatment as very painful, distressing, holding out false hope and always fatal sooner or later. I gave up reading about cancer.

But it was still inescapable. There were programmes about cancer on television which I now watched with morbid fascination. Some described cures by alternative methods such as changes in diet or visualization. They were tempting because they seemed to offer a way in which I could deal with the disease myself. But they didn't sound trustworthy. No, I placed my trust in God and in my belief that He was working through my doctors and guiding them in doing their very best for me.

On a television newscast I heard of an innocent shopper instantly killed when a lorry knocked her through a plate glass window. It made me feel thankful that I knew the probable circumstances of my death. That poor woman had never had time to say goodbye to her loved ones.

But things were catching up with me, too, and I was running out of time. The hospital was now certain of my donor. On May 11th I was once more admitted into the CMH, this time on the surgery ward to have my teeth taken out under general anaesthetic. The anaesthetist had only recently come into the army from Westminster Hospital where he had worked with transplants so that he knew just how carefully to monitor the drugs he would use on me. Evidence of God's complete care of me was rapidly piling up.

I came home on May 13th and went back again for chemotherapy from the 15th until the 17th—a whole week knocked off of the very few now remaining.

Only time for a few more flowers.

Though he was only four, I felt I must tell Cameron a little about what might happen. I felt he had a right to know and if I died, I did not want him to feel that I had betrayed him by going away and leaving him alone. I explained it as simply and undramatically as I could, but I used the words 'death' and 'die'. I told him that I did not want to leave him, but that if I died I would still be with him, looking down from heaven and loving and caring for him even though he couldn't see me. I told him that when Kirsty was old enough he must tell her this too. I must have made heaven sound a beautiful place because he wanted to go with me straightaway.

On June 5th a letter arrived from Westminster Hospital. It read simply:

> *Dear Nancy,*
>     *Just to let you know that we have got a definite date for your admission to Westminster Hospital on Friday, 19th June, for bone marrow transplantation on Saturday, 27th June.*
>     *See you soon.*
>                 *Yours sincerely,*
>                 *(signed) Dr. A. J. Barrett*
>
> *Dr. A. J. Barrett*
> *Senior Lecturer in Haematology*
> *Head of Department of Haematology*

There it was. In my hand. A one-way ticket to an unknown destination.

Though I had been expecting it, it was still a shock. At

the same time it was a relief to know that the months of uncertainty were over. I shoved it into a drawer. It must keep until tomorrow because that night George and I were going out for our last night alone together.

Some weeks before, I had entered a contest in our local paper, *The Aldershot Star* and had won first prize, dinner for two to a maximum of £20. When they learned of my circumstances, the paper generously offered a weekend in Paris instead – for two. I couldn't bear the idea of leaving my children now, even for so short a time so the newspaper extended the prize to a dinner for two worth £50 at Pennyhill Park in Bagshot.

It was an evening to see me through the many dark and lonely hours to come. We went early in the evening to enjoy the spectacular gardens before dining. It was a perfectly romantic setting and so far removed from family outings to the local chip shop as to seem in a different time and place, a place where we had just met and fallen in love. Fountains spraying water sprinkled soft music on the cooling summer air. All the flowers had a vibrant delicacy displayed as they were against the soft, deep green backdrop of towering rhododendrons. Only when it became too chilly did we come inside the Victorian country house for cocktails beside a warming log fire. The dinner was perfect in every respect and we made it last a long, pleasant time, a time alone and apart. It was like the night we first met over dinner in Tokyo nearly eight years ago. We never ran out of things to talk about. Happy things, about the past. The future was not even thought of as the evening, made mellow with Irish coffees, at last came to an end.

Like a reluctant child coming in from play, I woke the next morning and read the letter again. I handed it to George. Less than two weeks left.

A short visit to Westminster Hospital. My last blood test. Major Gravett and Dr. Barrett witnessed my will for me.

We were all in good spirits as at the beginning of an adventure. I resolved that there would be no turning back now. I know that it wasn't just coincidence that my very best friend was with me that day.

Nuria and I had taught at the same school, attended synagogue together and become like sisters while I was in Bangkok. Not good letter writers, in spite of our closeness, we had been out of touch since she had visited us in Nepal four years before. She surprised me with a phone call from London where she had bought a house to be near her children at boarding school in England though her home was still in Bangkok. I didn't know how much I needed her, but the Lord did. And here she was, holding my hand in the Haematology waiting room.

Mother arrived on June 11th laden with her own cases, boxes of gifts for the children and tins of chicken noodle soup and a rolled-up mattress for me. It reminded me of the sort of traveller one sees in Bombay airport. The mattress was a special foam sheet of an egg-crate design to make my long stay in hospital more comfortable. She brought a piece of real sheepskin as well!

On her first evening, after George and the children had gone to bed, she told me that God had given her a good feeling about me, a feeling He hadn't given her with Daddy. She knew without a doubt that I would be completely healed. She sounded so sincere and confident.

I didn't want to hurt her, but I remembered how she had said the same thing in her letter about Kirsty's birth. 'I'm glad *you* feel good about it,' I shouted somewhat angrily. 'You don't know how scary it looks from here. It's like standing blindfolded on a diving board, having to jump off and not knowing if there's any water or not in the pool.' Then I cried and the tears washed away my fear. In the few days I had left at home we didn't speak about it again.

These days passed all too quickly as I began making my

final preparations for departure. Flowers arrived, cards and letters from well-wishers, newspaper reporters and photographers and visiting friends. Anne Armstrong and a photographer came to do a feature story for *Soldier Magazine*. Dr. Watson came and I cried when I kissed him goodbye. As I took centre stage, it seemed that George receded into the background, one of the extras in the crowd scene. I didn't want it to be this way but I was swept helplessly along in the tide of all this activity.

On June 16th, Anne Armstrong had arranged an interview for me on British Forces Broadcasting. On the air, Tommy Vance asked me about my illness and the transplant and I made an appeal for the Haematology Research Fund at Westminster Medical School. It was very stimulating and all the staff were wonderfully kind. That evening we had our supper at the chip shop just as we had done nearly every Tuesday night since we had come to Aldershot. Mother was with us at this time. Otherwise we were pretending that nothing had changed.

On Wednesday I hired a projector and for the first time we saw the movies we had been taking since the children were born. On Thursday, my last day at home, George and I took Cameron to visit the Infant School he would start attending in September. George went back to work and Cameron and I had a little time alone together over a special treat of coca-colas. That night I gave him a cassette I had made of myself reading his favourite stories, saying a bedtime prayer and telling him and Kirsty goodnight.

On Friday, June 19th, hurried goodbyes to Anna and other friends were followed by last-minute packing. Early in the afternoon an Army ambulance came to take me away from all I loved most – my husband, my mother, my little children. I had asked them to let me go alone. I didn't want prolonged goodbyes nor awkward conversation during the journey. There was nothing left to say and I needed a small space alone. I needed time to prepare myself and asked them not to visit me until after the transplant procedure had begun.

I got through the goodbyes at the door with only a few missing heartbeats. With George and Mother, I only needed a kiss and an understanding look. Little Kirsty was spared understanding as she kissed me and waved, 'Bye, bye,' but Cameron broke my heart. Sensing our apprehension, probably feeling I was deserting him, he hid behind the door and refused to kiss me or tell me goodbye.

Very reluctantly I got into the front seat of the ambulance next to the driver. As he started to pull away I looked out and saw Cameron running across the grass towards us. I asked the driver to stop and I jumped out and ran to him and embraced his trembling little body. All the tears I had been so carefully repressing poured over both our faces as I promised him that I would be home soon. With a heavy heart I walked back to the ambulance, hoping I hadn't lied.

# Part Three

'Do not look forward to what might happen tomorrow; the same everlasting Father who cares for you today, will take care of you tomorrow and every day. Either He will shield you from suffering or He will give you unfailing strength to bear it. Be at peace, then, and put aside all anxious thoughts and imaginings.'

St. Francis de Sales

# 8

As the ambulance sped towards London, I tried to take in all the scenery. The rolling hills, the towering trees and rambling hedgerows, meadows dotted with sheep and the green freshness of an English summer's day. Would I see another? Perched jauntily on my head was Daddy's tweed cap. Underneath it was a pale face and an anxious heart.

What sort of journey was I on this time? What did one pack for eternity? Memories of people, places, experiences all carried in the suitcase of the soul. I wasn't travelling light.

Literally, too, I really moved in to the hospital loaded with all I thought I might want if I made it. I knew that I could be in isolation for a month or more and I was well prepared. To diminish any boredom I had brought several long books, a cassette recorder with tapes of classical music and Rod McKuen, a Scrabble game, graph paper to design a tapestry I wanted to make for Nuria and even a jigsaw puzzle in case I couldn't think. For my comfort I brought the mattress, the V-shaped pillow, my own bed pillow and chicken noodle soup and peanut butter. And for my inspiration, a collage of photographs of everyone in my family. Besides pictures of George and the children and Mother, there were photos of all my other relatives including Daddy and Aunt Lillian. These were the people who loved me and for whom I must get well. Finally, my worn paperback copy of *The Living Bible*; of all I brought the most necessary. Everything had to be new or able to withstand sterilization. Only my Bible could not be sterilized and I would have to read it through a plastic bag in the same way that I would any mail I might receive. Most of the scripture I needed I had memorized anyway.

Admitting myself into hospital, feeling perfectly fine and knowing that I was going to feel perfectly awful and perhaps even die, was the only brave thing I have ever done in my life.

After I had been admitted and settled into Edgar Horne Ward, I telephoned Nuria. She came to the hospital to see me and as I was not yet required for anything, the doctors allowed me to go out to dinner with her. Over a good dinner we laughed and chatted about our past travels and adventures together. We made a toast to future adventures together. This was just the sort of transition I needed between the afternoon of sad goodbyes and my first night alone at the hospital. I was back at the hospital by 7.30, in time to call home and tell the children and George and Mother goodnight. I spent the rest of the evening quietly praying as I finished Kirsty's tapestry. I had accomplished all of my own small tasks.

I wouldn't go into isolation until Tuesday but on Saturday the regimen to clean me up began. Every time I bathed I had to use a disinfectant soap. I had to use the same type of soap each time I washed my hands and face. Each time I ate or drank I had to immediately brush my teeth with a special toothpaste followed by a thorough rinse with an anti-bacterial mouthwash. I had to use an antiseptic aerosol spray for the insides of my ears and other inaccessible areas. I even had to swab out my belly button! I started taking septrin tablets against internal bacteria and began taking the dreaded Cyclosporin A. It had the taste and consistency of rancid olive oil. Bravely, I swallowed it

72

on its own. Back it came. I tried once more before I gave up and diluted it with a specially prepared chocolate and milk mixture. The milk had to be sterile.

The doctor from Radiotherapy came with a big pair of callipers and measured the thickness of my body in several places so that he could assess the dosage of radiation he would be giving me. He was very kind, but it made me feel now as though my body was from this time on completely out of my control, a piece of machinery.

Saturday afternoon I had an unexpected visitor. It was my bone marrow donor, Ian Kirby. I hadn't been sure if I wanted to meet him before the transplant. Supposing he liked me? Then he might feel very badly if I died. After he had been so kind in volunteering to save me, I didn't want that to happen to him. But there he was, standing beside my bed. The Good Samaritan, willing to give up his time, to risk a general anaesthetic and to suffer the discomfort of having marrow extracted from his bones for someone he had never met before. What could I say to such a person?

He fitted all the clichés – a knight in shining armour come to rescue me; tall, dark and handsome; the proverbial mysterious stranger. Any mystery was dispelled by his warmth, his modesty and his ready sense of humour during our brief conversation. He mentioned his job as a civilian with the Metropolitan Police Force and told me that he liked mountain climbing and football. We joked about whether I would take up these activities after the transplant.

It was only through writing to his mother much later that I learned that Ian is District Commissioner of the Islington Scouts Association, that he is a first class football referee not wanting to get involved with professional teams but sticking faithfully to the schoolboys' matches, and that he visits and collects money for mentally handicapped children. She wrote: 'Ian has always been a very caring person. I don't know if he is involved in other charities but I can assure you he always gives or helps if he can. You see, Nancy, as you say, Ian is very modest, he does not come home and tell you what he has done, a lot of it is hearsay from friends and neighbours. Also it would be very wrong of me to put Ian on a pedestal. That would never do. All I can truthfully say is that he is a very truthful, upright young man with very good morals and always ready to help anyone.' She assured me that Ian and everyone at their church was praying for my swift recovery.

On Sunday I was approached by a kind-looking woman in a long clerical gown. She wore a large gold cross and had sandals on her feet. Hesitantly I asked her if she was a lady priest as I had never met a deaconess before. Anne Richardson is an Anglican Deaconess ministering to the patients in Westminster Hospital. She invited me to the Communion service in the hospital chapel. I was grateful to go and find some Christian fellowship. I told her that Tuesday was the day of my transplant and Anne said that she would arrange the special service I requested for Monday.

Sunday afternoon the ward came alive with brightly-costumed fairies, medical students inviting mobile patients to attend the dress rehearsal of their production of Gilbert and Sullivan's *Iolanthe*. It was a surprisingly good production, an unexpected treat that brought back memories of my own acting and directing days. Coming back from the production we were led through a long, dark underground passage connecting the medical school and the hospital. The walls were lined with shelves containing thousands of medical files bearing the stamp 'Deceased'. I shivered as I wondered if my own file would soon be among these others.

Returning to the light and cheer on the Ward, I shook off this sense of foreboding and telephoned the family. I told them of my nice day and how well I was doing. But I was feeling a bit of my own 'stage fright'.

Monday morning the surgeon, Mr. Jones, came and showed me the Hickman's catheter he would be inserting into my body the next morning. It was about twenty-four inches long which rather shocked me. Mr. Jones assured me that once it was in place it would be painless. And best of all, there would be no more needles!

On Monday afternoon I went to the hospital chapel. There the hospital chaplain, Reverend Robert Clarke and Anne Richardson held a private Communion service for me. Reverend Clarke read Psalm 116 and then laid hands on me and anointed me with oil. My tears flowed freely as I promised them and myself and God that on the first Sunday I was able I would return to the chapel and read the lesson. From that moment on, I felt perfectly at peace.

On Tuesday morning the countdown to Day Zero began in earnest. I had a lovely long bath. My good Roman Catholic friend Myroulla had sent me a bottle of Holy Water and after I finished bathing, a bit unsure of how one was supposed to use it, I stood up and poured it over my head. It wasn't superstition. To me it was like a baptism and an affirmation of my faith in God's love and protection. I put on a clean white hospital gown. Like Isaac, I had gathered my own firewood and now I laid myself on the altar of my hospital bed and calmly waited knowing that God was watching over everything.


Drifting again. Floating in the familiar soft white clouds. The sky outside the windows spoke of late afternoon. I closed my eyes to the misty whiteness and slept again.

Only towards evening did the mist begin to evaporate. I felt a slight stiffness in my chest. I was in a strange room. On the window sill I could see my own books neatly arranged as if to say 'this is your home now'. I slept and woke again.

Now the sky was dark. The bedside lamp reflected dimly off walls of a murky mushroom colour, illuminating hideously-patterned drapes of brown and dusty rose. A soft voice welcomed me back to reality. Friendly brown eyes over a surgical mask. Her name was Donna McEntyre she told me, and she would be nursing only me throughout the transplant and the entire period of isolation. This was the isolation room. I closed my eyes to escape its gloomy atmosphere and slept again.

In the sunlight of Wednesday morning the room looked more cheerful — except for those awful drapes that would become far too familiar. They were spread over two adjoining walls of windows which overlooked an L-shaped balcony outside. There was a colour television set, a small refrigerator, two not-matching armchairs with vinyl covers, one dull green and the other dusty rose again. On a table stood a miniature cooker with two burners and a tiny oven. Another table and the shelves underneath it was laden with medicines, syringes and other medical paraphernalia. The usual bedside cabinet and tray on wheels completed the furnishings. It was rather like a clinical bed-sit.

Donna and I got a bit more acquainted. She was from New Zealand and had an accent it would take me sometime to master. But there wasn't time now.

It was time for the chemotherapy. The stiffness in my chest came from the incisions which had been made to put in the Hickman's catheter or line as it was now referred to. There was a small incision next to my right shoulder and another incision where about four inches of the line emerged from under my right breast. I was so relieved that the line had not been put in my neck after all! I watched with fascination as the line was uncapped and the doctor withdrew some blood with a syringe. Pinching off the end

76

of the line which had been swabbed with alcohol, he now connected the line to the IV bag containing the chemotherapy. That was two needles missed already. God bless Hickman, this line and I were going to be good friends!

This chemotherapy was much more powerful than any I had had before so I was slightly sedated in order to avoid too much sickness and vomiting. The chemicals were fed through the line along with other fluids so that my body could tolerate their harshness. There was no question of my trying to eat. The Cyclosporin A still had to be taken orally twice a day but apart from that I was left to doze during the treatment which lasted for the rest of Wednesday and all day Thursday.

On Friday when I was allowed a day of rest, George and Cameron came to see me. George had to be masked, gowned, booted and capped in order to come into my room. He even had to remove his shoes and wristwatch and wear plastic gloves. Anyone who came into the room had to first do this in a special cubicle outside the room and also wash their hands in disinfectant soap before putting on the gloves. Cameron was only allowed to look at me through the balcony windows where Donna held him up. For the few minutes that George stayed with me, Donna entertained Cameron by rolling his toy cars up and down the corridor. No doubt this is part of a nurse's training programme.

Saturday was officially Day Zero. The days were numbered so that close records could be kept of what to expect and what actually happened. I didn't know it at the time, but I was the first adult with an unrelated donor and the records might be of value in future transplants of this type.

On the morning of Day Zero, Donna bathed me and dressed me in a sterilized white gown, mask, cap, gloves and boots. I was then put onto a trolley well-padded with sterile

77

white sheets and blankets and wheeled down to Radiation. Westminster now had its own facilities for Total Body Irradiation (TBI), so a trip to the Royal Marsden Hospital was unnecessary. As it was Saturday the staff had shown great kindness by coming in on their own time and Donna chose to remain with me all day as well.

Over a period which lasted for eight hours I was given 950 rads (units of radiation), in forty minute doses. Between the doses my body was rearranged for me to give uniform exposure to all parts of it. The only other thing in the room apart from me on the trolley was a large clock on the wall. Watching it made the time go even more slowly.

The radiation room was very hot. Swathed as I was, all in white, I felt like an Egyptian mummy in a stifling tomb. I tried to occupy my mind by planning colour schemes for all the rooms of my fantasy dreamhouse. Fantasy because it could never withstand England's climate. Wrapping my mind in the colours of Eastern silks provided a foil against the whiteness surrounding me. A strong dose of pheno-barbitol helped to free my imagination.

The phenobarbitol was used as a defence against any sickness caused by the radiation, and only towards the end of the eight hours did I feel ill and vomit a little. Throughout the chemotherapy and the radiation I never became as ill as they expected. Again, I'm sure it was the Lord's protection.

If successful, the radiation would ensure that all of my own bone marrow was completely destroyed. Though I had dozed on and off during the day, the radiation made me very tired. When I was returned to my room, I slept until early evening.

While I had been in radiation, Ian Kirby had been in the operating theatre. Under a general anaesthetic long needles were inserted into some of his bones and about one litre of blood and bone marrow tissue was extracted. Refined, it

78

was brought to my room in an IV bag at about eight o'clock.

I felt another moment of stage fright as I watched the bag of rich dark red fluid being connected to my line. This was the last climatic scene.

Watching each bright drop fall into the line and flow into my body with the others, I repeated over and over again the precious words of Holy Communion – 'The blood of Christ, The body of Christ.'

Never had I felt such complete confidence.

# 9

Sunday. Day One. The period of waiting had begun and I was almost never left alone. Donna stayed with me from eight in the morning until eight at night when she was relieved by another nurse who watched throughout the night until Donna returned in the morning.

Each morning Donna had to clean the entire room. She washed down the walls with a spray disinfectant and scrubbed the floor and all the furniture with more disinfectant in boiled water painstakingly prepared in a small electric kettle in the room. Water was never taken from the sink. It was only used to empty the cleaning water and the drain was disinfected daily. Having to wear mask and gown all this work must have made her very uncomfortable in the unusually warm summer. The windows, of course, had to be kept closed for my protection. At night, the nurse on duty had to repeat this entire cleaning procedure.

When she had finished the room, Donna bathed me in bottled sterilized water using disinfectant soap and she washed what little hair I had left until it disappeared altogether. She watched me like a hawk to make sure I used all my disinfectant gels, sprays, mouthwashes and toothpaste. It wasn't that I minded these, I was just so tired that even using them was an effort.

I was beginning to catch on to her accent, but when she

said, 'We'll leave you here till later,' I was puzzled. As far as I knew there were no plans to move me out of this room. After several repetitions I was able to decipher what she had really said. 'We'll leave your *hair* till later.' We both laughed and it marked the beginning of our long friendship.

If I felt able to eat anything it was Donna who prepared it in my room. I was allowed nothing fresh except well-toasted bread. Any other food had to be tinned or frozen and eggs were strictly forbidden as they are full of bacteria. My crockery was kept immersed in the same solution used to sterilize babies' bottles and my cutlery was submerged in a covered dish of alcohol. After use they were washed in boiled water and returned to their sterile baths.

It was a long time before I even wanted to think about food. For most of the first week I was too tired even to look at television or try to read. Donna played my cassette of Chopin's piano *Etudes* over and over, and soothed by the music I slept most of the first week. My nourishment came through the line.

The only other part of my routine was a visit from the doctors, one in the morning to take blood from the line and usually one in the late afternoon just to see how I was feeling. I really appreciated these afternoon visits when we could talk like friends and the trouble they had to go to to make them as they, too, had to 'dress' every time they came into the room.

I had visitors during the week – George, Mother, Nuria and some of the staff from British Forces Broadcasting. I remember nothing of these visits except that it was nice to have them there. One of the patients I had met before I went into isolation came back to the hospital to see me with tins of asparagus and salmon! There were many unexpected treats like this and all through my illness people showed such kindness, even strangers. One man even interrupted his holiday in the south of England to come up to the

81

hospital and donate platelets for me. And most of all, I knew there were hundreds and hundreds of people praying for me.

On Day Seven was the Wimbledon Final between Bjorn Borg and Jimmy Connors. Just as the match was about to begin, Dr. Kendra came in to give me a transfusion of platelets explaining that he would stay with me to monitor my reactions (with one eye on the television screen, of course). Unable to locate any of the type of hydrocortisone I was usually given before platelets to prevent my getting chills, he used instead hydrocortisone saxonate. This type of hydrocortisone gave me the very painful sensation of having nails driven into my body, particularly in sensitive areas. I was frightened but it passed quickly and I was given the platelets. The platelets produced an even more frightening reaction. I felt as if there were iron bands around my chest and I could hardly breathe. I felt dizzy and saw spots before my eyes and the room growing black. I was sure I was finally dying and I was glad Mother was there so I could tell her goodbye. But this finally passed as well and, feverish and dizzy, I slept the rest of the day.

The next day I ate a little bit. On Day Nine my mouth felt too sore to eat and by the following morning my face was badly swollen and the insides of my cheeks were raw and bloody. I couldn't even swallow water and was reconnected to the drip. The doctors told me that it must be a reaction to the methyl-trixate I had been given to discourage *Graft vs. Host* disease (or GVH).

By Friday, Day Thirteen, the pain in my mouth was unbearable. I tried to escape in sleep and would wake to find the pillowcase soaked in blood. I tried to hold an image in my mind of the long, cool fingers of Jesus soothing my mouth and His words in a hymn kept running through my mind: 'I danced on Friday when the sky was black, but it's hard to dance with the devil on your back'.

I felt terribly depressed and I longed to see George but it wasn't his usual day to visit. I nearly asked Donna to call him and ask him to come. I didn't have to because he did come! I just held on to him and cried. To me it seemed another answer to prayer.

A telephone in the isolation room would have been such a help. In the awful loneliness and depression just hearing a loved one's voice is often sufficient comfort.

My mouth began to improve and my spirits lifted. I began to look forward to Sunday. George and Mother were bringing both of the children to see me so that I could be a part of Kirsty's second birthday celebrations.

I looked a bit like Popeye with my swollen jaw and I had to cover my completely bald head with a scarf. Looking so awful and with a tube coming out of my chest, still connected to the drip, I dreaded having the children to see me, but I wanted to see them so much. I wondered if I would frighten them or if they would even recognize that strange-looking person peering at them through the balcony windows.

They did recognize me and my appearance didn't seem to bother them at all! Through the window I sneakily passed the wrapped gifts I had brought into isolation with me for each of them and lightly touched their little hands. I longed to hold and kiss them. After they left, I cried. It was easier for me when the children didn't come. Seeing them caused too much distress and longing.

The long light days of summer blended into one another. The highlight of each morning was getting the results of the latest blood counts which continued to increase. I had bone marrow tests but was getting used to them though they were still painful. I picked out a wig that the NHS provided free of cost. I began to enjoy having visitors and I began to read again.

One of the books I had brought in with me was *The*

*Prophet* by Kanlil Gibran. Leafing through it at random I was startled to read these words: 'And when one of you falls down he falls for those behind him, a caution against the stumbling stone.' I suddenly realized that I had been chosen for a 'great and noble task' after all! Because my case was so experimental, whether I lived or died, the doctors would gain substantial knowledge that would benefit the treatment of all who followed me. Immediately I thanked and praised God for choosing me for this worthy task. I would do everything I could to justify His trust and confidence in me.

As if to reassure me, He sent me a dream-like vision. In it, I found myself in a place so beautiful and peaceful that it can only be described as Paradise. I was sitting in an open air theatre. The stage was empty. Daddy Bill, my grandfather, was sitting in a nearby seat and all the other seats were empty. He was staring at the empty stage and didn't seem to notice me. Then my Aunt Lillian came and led me away into a beautiful garden. Wearing a pink dress, she looked young and beautiful. The colours in the garden were more intense and clear than in real life. There were beautiful flowers and graceful trees. Even the many birds over our heads were of beautiful pastel colours – pink and turquoise, lemony yellow and pale lime. Then lying on our backs together we floated on a stream of warm water winding through the garden. It was strewn with flower petals. Though I don't remember all my aunt said to me, she was gentle and kind, with a radiant serenity. She asked me what I really wanted to do. I told her that I only wanted to be a mother to my children for another ten years or so, and she said, 'That's all right then'. With those words the dream dissolved.

(Only later did I wonder why Daddy Bill hadn't seen me and what he was waiting for. I still don't know.)

Except for the number of platelets, my blood counts continued to go up and I felt so much better as to begin experiencing boredom. The room seemed to have shrunk as I paced its confines trailing the dripstand which was on wheels. George and Mother came regularly. Mother's visits were getting longer, but George's were getting shorter. He did bring me treats of frozen lasagne and other things I requested, though.

Donna and I sometimes played Scrabble to pass the time. Every time I won I was delighted to see that my brain was still functioning normally. We gave up on the 5,000 piece jigsaw and donated it to another ward where it is probably frustrating someone else. It was far more interesting to discuss Donna's current boyfriends and social activities, a vicarious taste of the world outside the hospital.

One afternoon Ian Kirby dropped in for a visit and was so entertaining that Donna and I were still laughing after he had gone.

Finally, on Day Twenty-three my white blood cell count was high enough to risk exposing me to the outside world. On Day Twenty-four the doctors came into the room sans masks and gowns and announced that Isolation was officially over! Unfortunately this announcement was followed by yet another bone marrow aspiration, but I was too happy to mind – very much.

That afternoon George and Cameron came to see me. It was good to see George without a mask and wonderful to have Cameron actually sitting on my lap. And Donna was just as pretty as I imagined. I would be seeing less of her now as the regular ward nurses would be looking after me.

On the following Sunday, Day Twenty-nine, I felt able to keep my promise to the Lord. For the first time I would venture outside my room and go to the chapel to read the lesson.

I shunned the hospital dressing gowns I had been wearing every day and dressed myself in a long pink cotton dressing gown embroidered with tiny flowers. I had bought it in

Hong Kong where I wore it in hospital when Cameron was born. By the time I got my wig on and a touch of make-up I was now allowed, I was trembling with exhaustion. But borne along on my high spirits, dripstand in tow, I made my way to the chapel on the seventh floor.

The day was made even more special by having an organist for the service. That was a rare event. And though Psalm 116 was not the lesson for the day an exception was made so that I could read it instead. My hands were shaking but my voice was clear and my heart was full of promise as I read, 'I will worship you and offer you a sacrifice of thanksgiving. Here in the courts of the Temple of Jerusalem, before all the people'.

As the worshippers were leaving at the conclusion of the service, the organist played the haunting and familiar melody of *The Old Rugged Cross*. That had been Daddy Bill's favourite hymn. Curious, I thought, as I remembered the vision.

# 10

My jubilant morning in chapel made the blow that much more crushing when I was told the same Sunday afternoon that my platelet count had dropped from 71,000 to 31,000. The platelets or thrombocytes are cells in the blood which enable it to coagulate so that serious bleeding won't result from a cut or a wound. Normally, the platelet count ranges from 150,000 to 400,000. I couldn't share Mother's excitement when she described the rehearsal for the departure of the Royal Honeymoon train she had seen coming into Waterloo Station. Earlier, I had noted in my diary that I intended to be back at home in time to watch the wedding of Prince Charles and Lady Diana Spencer on television with the family. July 29th was only three days away. I pulled myself together and set a new goal. I *would* be at home to celebrate my birthday on August 17th.

The doctors discovered and began to treat a virus infection. Maybe that accounted for the drop in my platelet count. By the day of the wedding, my count had risen to 63,000.

As she was in England and so close to London, Mother was determined to participate as far as possible in the celebrations for the royal couple. Against the well-intentioned advice of both George and myself, she insisted on leaving Aldershot at six o'clock in the morning and joined the crowds lining the route the royal carriages would follow from Buckingham Palace to St. Paul's Cathedral.

I had crowds of my own drawn by the colour television set in my room. Extra chairs were brought in and any patients able to leave their beds were joined by nurses and auxiliary staff able to come in and watch between their duties. For a few happy hours the hospital atmosphere was suspended as everyone joined together in expressions of happiness for the royal couple. There was even a celebratory meal and wine in paper cups provided by the Queen herself.

Later in the afternoon Mother came into my now empty room and shared her exciting descriptions of all she had been able to see. We feasted on the tinned asparagus and salmon as we watched it all again on television. That night I suffered such an acute attack of indigestion that the doctor on duty wired me up to an electrocardiograph machine to make sure that I wasn't having a heart attack.

Although my platelet count had dropped back to 39,000 the next day, my spirits were buoyed up by being permitted to have a real bath in a bathtub. Until then the risk of infection had been considered too great and it had been thirty-seven days since I had had a proper bath. Dragging along my dripstand I managed to undress and manoeuvre myself into the tub. It felt so refreshing that almost an hour later, I hated to get out.

After the bath I felt so good that I put on a fresh dressing gown, my wig and a little make-up and even did my fingernails. Then, accompanied only by my dripstand, I went to the hospital library. Allowed 'used' books now, I checked out *Something Beautiful for God* by Malcolm Muggeridge and spent the rest of the day immersed in reading about Mother Teresa and her work. It was altogether a lovely day.

Each evening I was receiving transfusions of platelets, but by Saturday, Day Thirty-five, the count was down to

20,000. A visit from Kirsty saved me from feeling too depressed about it. It was only the second time I had seen her in six weeks and now I could hold her in my arms as she prattled and laughed in her baby voice. I gave her rides around the room on the base of the dripstand and she giggled and called it "Mommy's bicycle". By the time she left I felt good enough to go and have a short visit with the next patient awaiting a bone marrow transplant. I think I was able to transfer some of my renewed optimism to him.

The arrival of the next transplant patient meant that I would soon have to give up my private room with all its amenities. I had enjoyed being able to prepare some of my own food and eat it when I felt like eating it instead of being tied to the hospital's menu and mealtimes. I would miss this private retreat from the other patients and the activities on the ward and being able to watch the room's television set from the comfort of my bed. But 'graduation day' was upon me and it was time to face the world outside these safe four walls.

The day came sooner than I thought. I awoke on Monday morning, August 3rd, to find nurses on ladders taking down the curtains I hated so that they could be resterilized. As I sleepily got out of my bed, all my belongings were loaded onto it and it was pushed across the hall and onto the ward, my dripstand and me following breathlessly in its wake. Exhausted by this sudden flurry of activity I crawled back into my still-warm bed and dozed the morning away surrounded by the disorderly piles of my possessions on the floor, table, chair and the bed itself. My bed was separated from the others on the ward by a six-foot partition and the nurses kindly closed the curtains on all this clutter and let me rest until I felt able to cope with it. I was glad still to have this semblance of privacy and spent a pleasant afternoon arranging another temporary little 'home' for myself.

Besides making friends with some of the other patients, I could now enjoy more visitors and I was so appreciative of the efforts they made to come and see me. Anna came and another friend Margaret from Aldershot. Myroulla who had sent me the Holy Water came to see me from Thetford and another good friend, Pam, came all the way from the Isle of Wight. Nuria passed through London again, and my friend Lucy, on holiday from the 'States, visited me twice during her brief stay in London. Each one increased my determination to fulfil their wishes of 'get well soon'.

In spite of my platelets I felt well enough to begin extending my own get well wishes to other patients I met as I began to explore the third floor of the hospital. In the light of the suffering of others, my own illness seemed almost a blessing. I would either recover completely or die fairly quickly. But so many others I now came to know were faced with months or years of slowly progressing illnesses or conditions which could only be 'controlled' and with which they would have to learn to live for the rest of their lives. And yet, they all had concern and sympathy to spare for me. Me! who had been so blessed.

One of the very bravest patients I met was Jill Hicks, a frail but pretty girl sitting in a wheelchair in the third floor lobby. There were many other patients and visitors sitting in this communal area, but I felt particularly drawn to Jill. As I sat down near them, Jill and her visiting sister, Sue, introduced themselves and included me in their conversation. I have since learned that the Lord seems to make His followers known to each other.

Jill was only about twenty, a teacher who had had to give up her job when she began suffering from a debilitating illness called Motor Neurone Disease. Quite literally, she was wasting away physically, but beyond the doctors' expectations she was hanging on with an indomitable spirit made even stronger by her faith in Christ. She was in hospital now to have operations on her feet which might enable her to walk a little. Then, though she could easily live with her family, it was important to her to maintain her independence and she was determined to go back to her own flat and look after herself and intended to go back to teaching as soon as she was able. To all of us her very presence among us was an inspiration.

It was while bringing a book to Jill's bed on another ward that my ever-present dripstand introduced me to Rita and Maurice. The dripstand was tall and got caught on the curtain rail of Rita's bed. Maurice and I laughed about it and began talking as he disentangled me. He introduced me to Rita, his wife, whose bed was just across from Jill's and through frequent visits we all became friends. Rita and Maurice were Jewish so that we had a common ground. Often I visited with Rita in the evenings after Maurice had gone home and sometimes she asked me to read to her from the Psalms. Rita was suffering from cancer and as time went on I came to understand that it was so widespread throughout her body that there was no hope of a cure. Still Maurice always talked so cheerfully and positively to her about all the preparations he was making for her coming home where he and a nurse would look after her.

I enjoyed visiting these new friends but I still had many hours on my own to fill. I wished so much that I could use the time to write to all the people who had been so faithful in writing to me and in praying for me. They were sending me flowers now, too. In isolation I hadn't been allowed flowers as they carried a risk of infection. Now I couldn't even write thank-yous as my hands were so shaky from the Cyclosporin A. It was such a frustration. But I was learning to be patient.

Patient, too, with the continuing low platelet count. With almost daily transfusions of platelets, I was still making no progress. The doctors decided to try 'washing' my blood.

They would put me on the leukopherhesis machine and remove from my blood by a process of separation the immune complex and antibodies to platelets. Soon after they announced these plans to me, George came in and I told him about having my blood washed. With his usual dry wit he replied, 'Well, it's good weather for drying.'

We laughed, but I really dreaded the whole idea. I had been in hospital for forty days without a single needle and I was grateful, but I still hated the thought of even one. And then I thought of all the others who had been through this same process for me and I felt very small indeed.

On the morning that I was to have the leukopherhesis I turned to my Bible for a quick dose of courage. Opening it at random, I was met with this passage, I Peter 1:2: 'Dear friends, God the Father chose you long ago and knew you would become His children. And the Holy Spirit has been at work in your hearts, *cleansing* you with the blood of Jesus Christ and enabling you to please him. May God bless you richly and grant you increasing freedom from all anxiety and fear.' I was speechless to think that the Lord hadn't belittled my lack of courage but once again had given me just what I needed to overcome my fear!

In the leukopherhesis room I was placed on a bed lying nearly flat. My Hickman's line substituted for one of the two needles ordinarily used so that I only had a needle in one arm. Blood was drawn through the line and processed through the machine and returned via the needle in my arm. It was uncomfortable lying still for so long and I grew stiff and cold. The procedure took over four hours and the needle became increasingly painful. Then towards the end I got terrible chills. I was wrapped up in blankets and given hot tea, then wheeled back to the ward where I rested in bed for most of the rest of the day. I hoped that the platelet problem had now been solved.

The leukopherhesis had no effect on my platelet count

whatever. But any gloominess about my lack of progress was dispelled by the doctors' decision to disconnect me from my dripstand and allow me to go out-of-doors occasionally. The line was still intact and I was taught how to keep it viable myself with injections of heprinse.

The next morning, August 11th, as I was getting out of bed I automatically reached for the dripstand and was so happy not to find it there. I felt so free! I could walk about without looking for bumps in the floor or doorways that were too low, I could carry things in both hands. When George and Cameron came to visit me that day, I suggested we went out. I could hardly wait to feel the sunshine warm on my back, caressing my face.

My immunities were strong enough for me to be allowed fresh food and so we had our lunch out. What an assault on my senses – the traffic, the noise, the crowds and the colours – my head was spinning but I couldn't get enough. Everything was so vivid compared to the dim and quiet sterile world of the hospital.

I saw George and Cameron off at the bus stop and lingered outside in the warm air. A short stroll took me to the Christian book shop Mother had mentioned. There I bought C. S. Lewis's *Surprised by Joy*! I hoped it might give my still-interfering mind a 'logical' explanation for what had happened in my heart. But I didn't read it. Instead I bought a beautiful fresh peach and ate it in the hospital gardens gazing at the beautiful trees and flowers, the busy pigeons on the so-green grass. In spite of a small black cloud that had appeared on the horizon of my personal life, that night I slept deliciously.

It was just as well I had a good sleep because the next day was quite busy. First I had a bone marrow aspiration. Then a lot of blood was taken for further testing regarding the platelet problem. My donor, Ian Kirby, came up for a visit as he, poor soul, had been called in to give a large blood sample for testing too. As usual, he did so very cheerfully and we had a happy time together talking. I felt so indebted to him but there was nothing he would take in the way of thanks. All he wanted, he said, was for me to get perfectly well.

I had many other visitors that day so not until evening did I have time to consider that little black cloud and then it grew very much larger. George had brought with him the day before a sheaf of papers with house descriptions from estate agents. He planned to buy a house in Aldershot and look for a job there when he came out of the Army the following year. He saw no reason to wait until I could look at houses with him and didn't seem to consider it important that I didn't really want to live there. This caused the only real depression I had experienced in all this time in hospital. I didn't even know how to pray about this problem.

The next day the Lord sent Una, one of the ward nurses, to my rescue. She didn't ask me what was wrong. She didn't try to cheer me up or give me advice. She just held me and let me cry and cry. And though nothing changed as the days went by I began to feel better and better. Soon my inner-peace was restored and I could view the situation from the new perspective my born-again faith in the Lord had shown me. I could understand George's anxiety about coming out of the army and finding a good civilian job, to provide a home and food and clothing for us. He couldn't stop making plans whether I lived or died. Now I knew how to pray about it. I prayed that God would lift these burdens from George and give him the confidence of knowing that He had plans for George's good just as He had for mine.

On Day Forty-seven I was taken off steroids and on Day Forty-eight the doctors told me that they had at last discovered the cause of the platelet problem! Ian has a condition called Idiopathic thrombocytopenia or ITP which means that his marrow makes antibodies which destroy his own platelets. As Ian had compensated for this naturally all his life, the doctors felt that my system would do the same eventually. They even spoke of my going home soon and only coming in as an outpatient twice a week for transfusions of platelets.

I shared this good news with George the next day and he took it impassively. It was Kirsty with whom I shared my excitement as I played with her in the hospital gardens.

I didn't mind now that I had failed to meet my new goal of being home for my birthday. Mother came the day before my birthday and we had a wonderful celebration in my little cubicle. She had brought balloons and gifts and a splendid birthday cake which we shared with Donna and others.

The next day when it was really my birthday, all the doctors had sent me a card as had many of the nurses and other patients and all of my wonderful family in Omaha. How wonderful to know that so many people cared. It softened the hurt that I felt when George didn't come or even telephone.

During the afternoon I went for a walk to nearby Westminster Abbey. Looking at the beautiful old Abbey which had stood for nearly a thousand years made me feel very young. And in its shadow I felt the eternal presence of God. How could I ever thank Him for all the miracles He had bestowed upon me?

Later, when Dr. Barrett and some of the other doctors came in to wish me a happy birthday, I told them that it was not my forty-first birthday, but my FIRST birthday. For I had truly been born again both physically and spiritually!

# 11

Now that I had passed my birthday, the second goal I had set for being at home, I didn't know what date to circle on the calendar as my next goal. The expected twenty to thirty days in hospital had already become fifty-two. That wouldn't have mattered so much if I had been making progress, but I seemed to be in a state of suspended animation, neither slipping backward nor going forward, just standing still. No wonder George continued making plans without me. If I was growing tired of waiting, what must he feel?

It had been over a week since the ITP was discovered, but daily transfusions of platelets were having no impact on it at all. My platelet count continued to drop between transfusions.

There was no more talk of going home soon. Instead the doctors were talking about whether to try a course of a new form of immunoglobulin or whether to remove my spleen. I hardly cared which they chose as long as something was done.

The drug company Sandoz, of Switzerland, who also have invented Cyclosporin A, had manufactured a form of immunoglobulin thin enough to be given by transfusion. It was still in an experimental stage and had never been tried as a remedy for ITP, but Dr. Barrett felt that it might be of benefit. Because it was so terribly expensive, he had requested it through the Swiss Red Cross.

At least, if I wasn't progressing, others were. The operations on Jill's feet had been somewhat successful. Jill could stand up! There was general rejoicing among all of us who had grown to know, admire and care for her deeply. She was even being allowed home for the weekend. How could I be down when I was surrounded by so much evidence of God's love?

Mother's long visits were the highlight of my week. She came at least three times a week staying with me from ten o'clock in the morning until six o'clock in the evening and we never ran out of things to talk about. We had grown so close together, not just as mother and daughter, but as real friends. Now we were both daughters of the Lord, sisters in Christ. At the end of every visit we prayed together though it was Mother who spoke aloud. Without her nourishment I could never have grown so much in the Lord.

George came once or twice a week with one of the children, too, for an hour or so. Kirsty liked to get in bed beside me and be cuddled. Cameron liked to take my blood pressure with the sphygmomanometer which he had even learned to pronounce, and he was delighted when Dr. Kendra let him help change one of my IV bags. I hated seeing them get so used to this routine. I wanted them to have a normal mother who lived at home and tucked them into bed every night.

It was the hours between visits that were so long. I still could barely decipher myself the notes I tried to make in my diary, so writing letters was still out of the question. Besides, what 'news' did I have to write about? I couldn't manage a tapestry needle either. I had read every book in the hospital library about India and the Far East. Though I am probably the world's worst knitter, I asked Mother to get me some wool and a pattern and I started making a cardigan for Kirsty. At least I could hold on to the large knitting needles.

Probably because I did not feel physically ill this position of marking time was so dispiriting and tedious. I had already seen so many patients come and go that I couldn't help feeling left out or left behind.

Only Rita remained, though I could see that she was leaving, too. She was becoming more distant and vague as they increased her doses of pain-killing drugs. Sometimes she failed to recognize me though I continued to stop by her bedside almost every night before I went to bed myself. I longed to be of comfort to Maurice but he would still not acknowledge openly that Rita was dying.

I prayed for Rita. She had such a sweet spirit. Was I the only one to see a glowing light in her face and around her bed? In John 14:6 Jesus says, 'No man cometh unto the Father, but by me.' Rita was Jewish but I couldn't believe that God would deny her eternal life; Jesus couldn't have meant that. I longed for understanding. I prayed for an answer.

Ten days after my birthday, Mother began to talk of going back to America. In September Cameron would begin attending Infant School fulltime and an exception had been made for Kirsty so that she could attend Queen Mary's Nursery School for the entire day although she was more than ten months under the usual admittance age of three. Mother couldn't be of much further use and decided to return home. She hated to leave me, of course, but she had come to know all my doctors well as they answered her many questions over the weeks, and she was confident she would be leaving me in safe hands. We discussed this over lunch at an outdoor café in Covent Garden, my most adventurous outing to date. It made it even more obvious that there was very little more she could do for me by staying on. Though I realized with a stab of pain in my heart just how much I would miss her, it was the time for letting go.

I was very tired by the time I got back to Horseferry Road late that afternoon. I had a raging headache and no appetite for my dinner. I only thought it was my body's response to the tiring excursion, ample lunch and my sadness at the prospect of Mother's leaving.

The doctors knew otherwise. The following day my symptoms persisted and I also had a temperature. I was sent down to X-ray for an upper GI, gastro-intestinal X-Ray, which confirmed that I had picked up an intestinal infection, probably in hospital. I had managed to walk down to the X-Ray Department but felt so weak and dizzy that I had to be wheeled back on a trolley, though it embarrassed me terribly after I had told everyone I wasn't really sick. After a few days on antibiotics I felt well again.

I felt very fine. The Swiss Red Cross were going to send the Sandoz Globulin free of charge. Mother felt more relaxed about leaving with this news and went ahead and booked her ticket to leave one week later. The doctors said I could spend a day or two at home before she left. George said only that he didn't think that was a good idea. I couldn't explain my tears to anyone.

George and Cameron came to visit me on the Saturday before Mother's Monday departure. We took Cameron to the park and watched him play. We seemed to have nothing to talk about and it was almost a relief when they left. The sense that we were drifting farther and farther apart with each passing day increased. I felt unutterably sad.

On Sunday Mother and I began our last day together by taking Communion in the hospital chapel. She had brought tuna fish sandwiches with her, a mutual favourite, and we were going to have a picnic over by the Thames. On impulse we took the boat trip to Greenwich instead and spent a really beautiful afternoon together until it was time to say goodbye. Then the tears flowed freely as we had our last prayer together and the elevator doors slid between us.

For the last three months we had been closer together than in all our lives before.

On Monday morning I received a tender little greeting card with a loving farewell note Mother had written and mailed earlier. She had always done such thoughtful things. There was some money in the envelope as well. That afternoon I went out and spent the money on a Children's Bible for Cameron and Kirsty. When I came home, I vowed to myself, I would teach them about Jesus' wonderful love and how He saved and healed me. And I would try to be as wonderful a mother to them as my mother was to me.

The days seemed even longer now. I still saw Donna from time to time and even Dr. Watson from Aldershot surprised me with a visit. But it was meeting Mary Gallagher that helped most to fill in the gap left by Mother. Mary was a Haematology patient of long standing. She was about my age and had been in and out of hospital since she was only nine. Mary has sickle cell anaemia. It produces recurrent attacks of fever and pain described by the term 'crisis'. In order to stave off these crises Mary had to have a complete blood change about every six weeks. I simply couldn't imagine a life dependent on transfusions and needles and my own problems paled in comparison. Yet, of all the patients I met, Mary was the most cheerful.

Through Mary I became part of a group of 'regulars' at the hospital. After visiting hours we would take it in turns to make tea and toast in the hospital kitchen and stay out in the lobby chatting. There, Tim Murphy, a garrulous Irishman kept us laughing with his never-ending string of humorous stories. He even made us forget that he had just about exhausted the possibilities of treatment by dialysis and that if a kidney donor wasn't found for him soon he couldn't go on much longer.

Now, at last, I was beginning to ask, 'Why me?' I had never even thought of asking it when I was told I had leukaemia. I was asking it now because I couldn't understand why the same miracles did not seem to be happening for Jill, for Tim, for Mary and for Rita. After our evenings of tea and toast I still went to tell Rita goodnight. More and more now I found her already asleep.

As I approached her bed one night, I thought Rita was already asleep and I was rather relieved because I was sleepy, too. Then she opened her eyes and smiled at me. She looked truly beautiful and more alert than I had seen her for a long time. She asked me to bring her the telephone. I tried to discourage her as it was about ten o'clock but she insisted and I couldn't bear to refuse. In spite of the drugs, she dialled the number without any trouble. As I left I heard her telling Maurice how much she loved him and saw the tears glistening on her cheeks.

In a short while I returned to collect the telephone. Rita was calm. She asked me for some grapes. I searched the kitchen's refrigerator to see if Maurice had left some for her as there was nothing beside her bed. There were none in the refrigerator nor could any of the nurses find any anywhere. Nor could I tempt her with anything else. Though I was sure she had no appetite, she persisted in her request for grapes.

There was nothing I could do except say a short prayer with her and tell her goodnight. With a heavy heart I walked back to my own ward.

As I came to my bed I saw a brown paper bag on my table. I hadn't put it there. Curiously, I opened it and inside I found – a beautiful bunch of grapes!

'My husband brought those,' the patient in the bed across from me called, 'but I'm not allowed fruit. I thought you might like them.'

I could hardly comprehend it as I thanked her. It wasn't a bag of apples or bananas or pears. It was *grapes*.

My weariness vanished as I hurried to take the grapes to

Rita. She ate only one but I could see the bliss on her face. She held a second grape as she fell asleep in contentment.

I was contented, too. I knew that the Lord had answered me, and that He loved Rita. A few days later Rita died.

# 12

At last on September 18th, Day Eighty-four, the Sandoz Globulin arrived! It had been twenty days since I was told it would be coming, and the doctors had told me that it would probably take another week or two after it was given to me to see what the results were. It did nothing to dampen my once again soaring spirits. At last we would be *doing* something after all this time of just standing still. Excitedly I told the tea and toast group my good news that Friday night. The treatment would begin on Monday.

George surprised me by coming earlier than usual Saturday morning and he finally caught me with nothing on my bald head. I was so embarrassed! I must have reminded him of a boiled egg because he said, 'I've already had my breakfast. Next time I'll bring a spoon.' My embarrassment dissolved as we both laughed together and I told him my good news. 'Maybe things will be all right when we're together again', I thought.

I sailed through the weekend daydreaming of how the immunoglobulin would solve the platelet problem and I would be home and well and happy with my children and with George. In the chapel on Sunday I prayed earnestly for the success of the treatment. If I didn't feel much like eating, well it must be because I was so full of anticipation.

My platelet count on Monday morning was 12,000. Once that had been established, my Hickman's line was again connected to the dripstand and over a period of an hour or so I was transfused with twenty-four grams of the Sandoz Globulin. Other patients stopped by my bedside to wish me well and Mary told me she was praying for me and so was Father Murphy, the Catholic chaplain for the hospital.

By Tuesday morning the platelet count was 33,000 and my hopes rose with it. Then I was given another twenty-four grams of the immunoglobulin. Reporting my new count the other patients celebrated with me over our tea and toast. On Wednesday morning the count had dropped slightly to 30,000, but the doctors told me they were still confident that the drug was working as the count was stable even though I hadn't had a transfusion of platelets for nearly a week. I then received the third dose of twenty-four grams. That night Mary and the others gave me their encouragement and I began to realize how much I would miss them when I finally got to go home.

Thursday's count was 50,000. I was given the final dose of immunoglobulin and Dr. Barrett told me that if the count continued to rise, he could see no reason why I couldn't go home that very weekend. After all this time, I could hardly take it in. Going home! Was it too good to be true, Lord? Have you answered my prayers and the prayers of so many others for me yet again? I was sure He had.

Donna wanted to help me celebrate, too. Friday afternoon she took me out to tea at Harrods. I wished I had more appetite for all the wonderfully tempting confectionery spread before us. I loaded my plate and so did Donna and we chatted happily as she demolished hers and I picked at mine. I was probably just too excited about going home tomorrow.

On the way back to the hospital I bought some sausage rolls, cold meats, cheese and cakes. The isolation room was empty. Two bone marrow transplants had come and gone successfully since I had been in. They both had aplastic anaemia and related donors. I sneaked my goodies into the room and that night while the others were making the tea and toast, I used the little oven in the isolation room to heat the sausage rolls and surprised them with my little celebration feast. Everyone was so happy for me. How I would miss them all, especially Mary!

My going home on Saturday was dependent on the platelet count and I wasn't disappointed. It had risen to 73,000!

I called George, then hurriedly packed my things and got dressed. While I waited for him I went around the wards telling everyone goodbye, not without a few tears. I didn't need lunch because I would be eating at home. I gave Esther, another member of the tea and toast brigade, my still almost full jar of kosher dill pickles.

It seemed like a dream going home with George, and the children accepted me as naturally as if I'd never been gone. I telephoned Mother and when I told her I was speaking to her from home, she was ecstatic. So was I.

The weekend was relaxed with dear George dressing and looking after the children and doing all the cooking. I tired easily and this was augmented by the frolicking playfulness of the children. I just wasn't used to all their noise and confusion after my orderly hospital routine. Still I loved every minute of being with them and hated it when their bedtime seemed to come so soon.

In the quiet of the evening when George and I were alone, we simply watched television. After a brief bit of conversation about the children it seemed we had nothing else to talk about. I was disappointed but I reasoned that it was quite natural as we had led quite separate lives for the last few months. It had been four months since our dinner at Pennyhill Park and that was the last time we had really talked to each other.

On Monday George walked me up the steep hill to the

Cambridge Military Hospital once again for a blood test. I was all smiles inside as I watched the doctor prepare his needle to take a sample from my vein, and I laughed as I pulled the end of my line from my bra where I kept it safely tucked away and showed him how to use it. The blood counts, including the platelets, were all quite satisfactory. The short walk to and from the hospital made me too tired for lunch. I just had a bath and then a nap as George had taken the day off.

On Tuesday George went back to work. The children were both at school. The house seemed so quiet and empty as I explored it alone. I felt just like the 'fish out of the sea' and almost missed having my temperature and blood-pressure taken and all the other hospital disciplines that had become an expected part of my daily life for so long. Certainly, I missed the company of Mary and Donna and my other friends at Westminster.

After all my enforced 'rest' I was actually looking forward to doing some real housework and rather disappointed that George had managed so well that there was very little to do. As I happily pottered about the house doing little bits here and there, I was thinking how pleased he would be to be relieved of all the extra chores my being away had imposed upon him. That night when George returned from work with the children at half past four, they all took off their coats and George went straight to the kitchen and started preparing dinner. I had planned to make dinner myself that night at our usual time of six o'clock. Surprised, I followed him into the kitchen and began helping him but I only felt useless and in the way. He had established his own very efficient routines. Well, I thought, it's bound to take time for us to get used to one another again and I left the kitchen and played with the children until George announced that dinner was ready.

Somehow I managed to get through the rest of that week

and the next doing whatever I could manage in the house and for the children. I made it back up to CMH for another blood test and was very pleased to learn that my platelet count was now 158,000. I had been a bit worried as now I was eating less and less and suffering from cramps and diarrhoea and my hands and feet felt a little numb. The doctor at CMH gave me some tablets and I felt it would soon clear up. I decided it wasn't worth telephoning Westminster about it.

But the illness persisted and the following Monday George called a taxi to take me up the hill and I was admitted to the CMH yet again. I even had the same room. Between the attacks of stomach cramps and diarrhoea, all I wanted to do was sleep and sleep and sleep.

I was due for my first check-up at Westminster on Wednesday but I asked the nurse at CMH to put it off until Friday. I was sure I'd feel better by then. On Friday morning the Army ambulance took me back to Horseferry Road. An Army nurse helped me walk down the stairs to Haematology for my check-up. The next thing I knew I was being wheeled on a trolley. I saw the words 'Edgar Horne' flash past and remember thinking, 'I'm safe now.'

It was October 16th, Day One Hundred Twelve.

# 13

I remember the shocking pain of a lumbar puncture and a bone marrow aspiration and that it was Dr. Joshi who performed them. I remember being moved into the room where Tim Murphy had been and how ominous it seemed when they told me Tim had died of cardiac arrest only a few days after I had gone home in September. That's all I remember until I finally became fully conscious again sometime during the first week of November.

The Hickman's line had kept me alive as I laid curled up in a foetal position, cocooned in blankets. Now I emerged with reluctance. The doctors welcomed me back with relief. Later, they confided that they really had thought they were going to lose me. Only my complete trust in God sustained me as I now awoke to find myself faced with a nightmare of tortuous testing as the doctors struggled to come up with the correct diagnosis. The symptoms were very much like *Graft vs. Host* disease, but they couldn't be sure without more detailed analysis.

I felt absolutely miserable – weak, tired, feverish and far, far more nauseous than I had ever felt with the chemotherapy. My mouth was sore and burning and even the thought of eating or drinking sickened me. Sweet Dr. Halil sat by my bedside for nearly half an hour as she gently and patiently helped me get down forty tablets crushed in milk since this drug could only be given orally.

My weight had dropped to just over six stones, a loss of 25 pounds and everyone was encouraging me to eat, but I just couldn't. I managed to sip at this more out of appreciation for their efforts than any real desire for it. I am sure it was God who once again sent Nuria to me.

On an unplanned stop in London, Nuria had telephoned the house and learned that I was back in hospital. Now she was not only here with me, she had brought me a tin of that chicken noodle soup! Only the Lord could have led her to do that. She asked a nurse to prepare it and mainly for Nuria's benefit I had a few spoonfuls, appreciating her thoughtfulness much more than her gift. But the soup did taste so good and it was my first step towards eating again.

George came up once or twice a week and as I began to feel up to it, he brought me MacDonald's milkshakes. Nuria came nearly every evening as she extended her stay to be near me as well as her children at boarding school not far from London. And her children sometimes came to see me at the weekend. Every time she came, Nuria brought more tins of soup, but I didn't tell her my bedside locker was full of unopened tins of it. She stopped bringing soup and she started bringing milkshakes, too. I accepted the milkshakes from George and Nuria with gratitude and the nurses helped distribute all the surplus.

Emaciated and bald, looking and feeling dreadful, I was glad not to have any other visitors. I still slept most of the time and could feel myself slipping into the valley of the shadow of death.

There was a long day's session of barium X-Rays of my oesophagus, stomach and intestines. Swallowing the awful liquid increased my nausea even more. I dozed fitfully between the sessions on the X-Ray table.

I spent another awful day with a Crosby capsule. This was a small metal sphere on a long plastic cord which I had to swallow, a difficult task, causing me to gag as my throat was still raw and sore, even more so due to the previous barium meal. After several attempts I managed to keep it down. Now, suspended by the cord the capsule should make its way down to my stomach. It's progress was followed by an X-Ray every twenty minutes or so. Hour after hour I had to struggle against my body's impulse to vomit it up as the capsule refused to reach the desired position. Once it did, by pressing the apparatus at the other end of the cord the capsule would open and clip off and enclose a small piece of tissue as it snapped shut. Then it would be pulled up and out and a biopsy could be done on the tissue. After seven agonizing hours the capsule had still not found its goal. Nuria had come by then and helped me to persuade Dr. Joshi to take a snip where it was and take it out. Not satisfied with the results they obtained, I then had to suffer the indignities, to say nothing of the discomfort, of a rectal biopsy.

At last it was concluded that I did not have *Graft vs. Host* disease. That, at least, was a great relief. I had candida, a fungal parasite, all through my digestive system. Everyone normally has a minute quantity of this fungus, but because of my low immunities my candida had got completely out of hand.

Even though the diagnosis was finally made and real treatment had begun, physically and even spiritually I was at my lowest ever. I was convinced that I was going to die. I was absolutely certain that the doctors and nurses were only telling me reassuring things in order to hide that truth from me. As I became more dependent and withdrawn, their support and encouragement increased, but still I would not believe them.

The entire staff of the Haematology Department sent me a cheerful but sympathetic greeting card. Busy nurses popped in during their free moments in an attempt to cheer me. Dr. Kendra even interrupted his busy schedule to sit by my bedside for over an hour, holding my hand and soothing me, trying to convince me that I really would feel better soon. Pauline, a young trainee nurse prayed beside my bed and kissed me gently on the cheek. The love of Christ shone through her and through all those who wanted me well. I only longed for heaven and the cessation of this noxious, never-ending feeling of illness.

As George was leaving after a visit one afternoon when I was feeling at my very lowest, I couldn't help crying a bit. 'Say a little prayer for me,' I wept. There was a harsh edge to his voice as he answered with, 'You know I don't believe in that rubbish,' and he turned quickly and walked out of the room.

At first I just lay there stunned. Then I cried and felt sorry for myself and for him. I stopped crying as my hurt turned itself into resolve. I must get well! I must stay with my children and teach them of the reality of God and of the wonderful love He has for each of them. So much love that He sacrificed His son Jesus to save us and show us how to live. So must I, for now, sacrifice the peace of Heaven and show my children how to live and walk in the way of the Lord!

I didn't tell George this. I didn't tell anyone. I just picked up the scattered pieces of my spiritual armour and with the confidence that 'His loved ones are very precious to him and He does not lightly let them die,' I resolved that I would live.

On the 28th of November George brought Cameron and Kirsty to see me. Kirsty gave me an amusing account of 'Baby' school where she said she had 'bean pies' and 'baby pudding' for lunch. And Cameron gave me a picture he had drawn at school of me in a hospital bed and a touching bouquet of ragged paper flowers he had made for me. Once more I began to dream of going home for another Christmas.

The candida was slow to surrender its hold on my body, the awful nausea persisted and there were several setbacks, but I held on to my dream and gradually I began to improve.

Nuria and her children came to say goodbye to me on the 12th of December. They were going back to Bangkok to celebrate Channukah and she promised she would see me in January – at home.

I thought I would be lonely in my separate room, but then Valerie came in the door. She was another Haematology patient and was going to have a Hickman's line put in. She was a bit nervous about it so Dr. Barrett had told her to come to see me and see what the line was like. Like me, Valerie was wearing a small gold cross and after we had finished talking about the line, we talked about the Lord. We became close friends sharing our hopes and our prayers.

Valerie would have to stay in hospital for Christmas, but she counted it a blessing to be able to share this Holy day with others far more lonely. On the 22nd of December I was told that I could go home, not just for Christmas but to stay!

The doctors also chose that moment to tell me that I was probably the oldest bone marrow transplant with an unrelated donor, possibly the only person cured of leukaemia by this method and certainly the world's longest surviving bone marrow transplant with an unrelated donor! It was only Day One hundred and seventy-nine, less than six months since the transplant, and though I was happy for myself, it made me sad to think that others had not survived for even that long. More than ever I realized God's own guidance was responsible for my miraculous healing. It was even one of the Hindu doctors who, getting things in the correct order, said, 'Thanks to your prayers and our skill, you are well.'

112

On December 23rd I went home to celebrate the birth of His Son, my saviour Jesus, with a heart full of gratitude.

On Mother's Christmas card to me she had written: 'In 1970, I felt very burdened for your salvation. For ten days I fasted and prayed asking for guidance in how to be a witness to you. On the ninth day I had a vision. In it, I saw myself walking down a long corridor. All the doors I passed on either side of the corridor were closed, and to me they seemed to represent the closed doors of your ears, your mind and your heart. But the last door, on the left side, was standing open and from it shone a great beam of light. To me, it meant that someday you would be saved.'

On the third floor of Westminster Hospital, at the far end of the corridor, my room was the last one on the left.

# Epilogue

*'I shall be telling this with a sigh*
*Somewhere ages and ages hence:*
*Two roads diverged in a wood, and I—*
*I took the one less travelled by,*
*And that has made all the difference.'*

Robert Frost
'The Road Not Taken'
Holt, Rinehart & Winston
(Jonathan Cape Ltd., London)

*'. . . but when you don't have faith,*
*you don't see the miracles.'*

Isaac Bashevis Singer
*The Penitent*
(Farrar, Straus, Giroux, New York, 1983)

# Epilogue

On a day I cannot number, a day when I was still in isolation, I read again Psalm 116. It includes these words: 'I will worship you and offer you a sacrifice of thanksgiving.' Though I had never written anything in my life, without hesitation I made this commitment to the Lord: if I survived the transplant, I would write a book telling others of His goodness to me.

I did not make this promise in an attempt to bargain with the Lord. And I know that He did not make it a condition for my healing and salvation. In answering the question, 'Why me?' Why did God choose that *I* should live? I believe that He healed me for no other reason than that He loves me. If He does not heal some others, perhaps it is because He loves them even more (Isaiah 57:1-2). This book is simply an expression of my thanksgiving to Him and, I hope, an encouragement to others who suffer.

With the last chapter you have read, I thought I had fulfilled that commitment. Then the Lord told me, 'The story is not yet finished.'

It is true. On December 25, 1981 I felt that I had reached the mountaintop both physically and spiritually. It would be wrong of me to leave you feeling that I had. So it was when once I went climbing in the foothills of the Himalayas. The going was very rough for a complete novice, but with the goal clearly in sight going up the initial slope was fairly easy and I was carried along by my enthusiasm. But as the path got steeper and harder to discern among the undergrowth, it became a gruelling task to force my aching leg muscles to carry me on. Always looking up I would see a peak just before me that, standing alone against the sky, seemed to be the top of the mountain. But just as I would reach that peak, I would discover another higher one looming behind it. And so it is with my story. I must keep on climbing.

Just as on those lower slopes, in the hospital, free from my worldly responsibilities and daily routine tasks, there was plenty of time for prayer and meditation. Among strangers there was no interference with nor opposition to my beliefs. I led a cloistered sort of life in which it was easy to be a Christian. Once at home I faced the challenge of the higher slopes, of learning to practise this faith and the change of habits and temperament it required in the face of physical weakness and lack of energy, of recurrent illnesses, of time consumed in never-ending household tasks, of sometimes very naughty children who tried my patience to the limit and of an unbelieving husband who seemed no longer to understand me.

Amidst this sort of undergrowth it is often difficult to find and follow the right path and I do not always succeed. But I find my blessed Lord never condemns my failure but is always ready to lead me back to the way when I call upon Him. He didn't teach us to pray for enough bread to last for a week or a month or a lifetime but to ask only, 'Give us this day our daily bread'. And as we turn to Him each day, so the bread is always fresh and sufficient for our needs.

Physically, the climb has been arduous but much progress has been made.

In January 1982, the Westminster Hospital requested blood samples from George and the children so that by a process of elimination they could reassess some of the factors in my blood. I hated to see my children have even one needle, but it cleared one doubt which still lingered. The leukaemia was neither hereditary nor contagious. Daddy's having acute erythro leukaemia and my having acute myeloid leukaemia was entirely coincidental. Though the children had been exposed to both of us and it could even have been beginning in me while I was carrying Kirsty, neither of the children was affected in any way.

For a long time I continued having debilitating stomach aches as my digestive system recovered from the effects of the candida. They slowed down my progress in taking up my household tasks, and as I didn't seem reliable, George had a good excuse for carrying on alone.

Then, in March, I had to stay in hospital overnight as the Hickman's catheter was finally removed. Though it had caused a trauma when the line burst one night in December, a clever houseman had managed to repair it and it had been a faithful friend for nine months. Now it was back to the needles. A few days later George and I attended Cameron's Mother's Day programme at school. All the children made picture posters of their own mothers bearing captions that began with the words, 'I love my mummy because . . .' Most followed with things like 'she cooks my favourite food', or 'she washes my clothes'. Cameron's said, 'I love my mummy because she cuddles me.' At least, if I wasn't doing much, I was doing what was most important.

The stomach aches finally ceased and I did more and more of the other things too. Each day brought a new sense of achievement as I marvelled at all I was now able to do. I caught myself saying to myself things like, 'This is *me* carrying all this shopping! Oh, thank you, Jesus!'

But in June, just one week short of the first anniversary of the transplant, I was again rushed down Horseferry Road to Westminster Hospital with a serious bronchial and ear infection. What in an ordinary person would be little more than a cold, my immune system could not yet cope with. Any illness could attack and overcome me within hours, ja lesson I have had to learn many times over. Still, my week's stay in hospital was beneficial in enabling me to have more and longer times alone with the Lord than I could manage at home and in reminding me of the wonderful changes He had brought about in my life just because I had been so very ill.

Everyone on earth has limitations. There are no exceptions from this and there is no 'fairness' in their distribution. Illness is not caused by God. He does not use it to single out and punish anyone. Illness is only one of the limitations imposed upon us by our choice to live outside of Eden. But with the transforming power of God's love and acceptance, all of us can live fully within our limitations. Even in illness. In fact, it is so often through our own suffering that we are allowed to glimpse the suffering of our Lord, to understand more deeply the significance of His sacrifice made for us and of His power to sustain us through adversity that it is almost a privilege to suffer. And if we come to Him with the faith of a little child, He will 'kiss it and make it better'.

After coming home in June I noticed that my muscles were becoming increasingly tender so that the slightest touch caused pain and that at the same time they were becoming stiff and I was getting searing cramps more and more often. So, in August I was again back in the Westminster for a few days for a muscle biopsy. Under a general anaesthetic slivers of muscle tissue were taken from my left arm and leg. The results were not dramatically conclusive but seemed to indicate a form of *Graft vs. Host* disease in which, put simply, my new lymphocytes had taken a dislike to my muscles and were attacking them. I was put back on steroids and Cyclosporin A and the condition is now stabilized and somewhat improved.

With only occasional days of feeling a bit off, I did well until November, when again with no warning, I was struck down, this time with severe septicaemia, or blood poisoning. I was in Intensive Care for four days with a tube, this time in my neck and without the benefit of an anaesthetic, but I was not frightened. I had learned to pray only, 'Father, if it be thy will'.

There have been other attacks of illness though these are becoming less and less frequent and far less severe. I mention these only in the hope that it will encourage others not to give up in the face of their own setbacks. Always, my illnesses have brought me closer to God.

One night during a stay in hospital, I woke up in the dark hours of the morning, perfectly clear-headed for the moment, with two lines of poetry in my mind as firmly as if they had been printed there. They were not my own words and I had never heard them or read them anywhere. Without thinking, I scribbled them down in the dark on a paper towel on my bedside table and immediately went back into a deep sleep. In the morning I wondered if I had been dreaming, but there was the paper towel with these words on it!

*'Of food and drink the creature sings*
*And God says, "Oh, my own sweet thing". . .'*

Through the following days and nights more words came to me at odd moments until I knew, at last, that the dictation was finished. This was the complete poem:

*Of food and drink the creature sings*
*And God says, 'Oh, my own sweet thing,*
*My body is the living earth,*
*The bread you've eaten since your birth.*
*And all its fruits, My blood, the wine.*
*You are the branch, I am the vine.'*

*In dark despair the creature sings*
*And God says, 'Oh, my own poor thing.*
*To cleanse your soul no water may.*
*My tears alone wash sin away.'*

*In anguished pain the creature cries.*
*'My precious one, don't weep,' God sighs.*
*'In My Word your healing lies.*
*Who suffers for My sake, never dies.'*

*Of home and hearth the creature sings*
*and God says, 'Oh, my cherished thing,*
*My heart's your hearth, My arms your home.*
*You never need feel all alone.*
*With tender love I ever embrace*
*My whole dear, sad, sweet human race.'*

The words I had written were not mine, but God's I believe. Words that defined and expressed what I truly now believed. My doubting mind became quietened at last.

George got a very good job when he came out of the Army, and I couldn't be more pleased with the house which we chose together. But in so many ways we are still strangers. It takes a great deal of love, patience and understanding to close the gap created by such a long illness and separation.

Because a medical breakthrough had been made in my case, there was a lot of publicity and attention given to me. Though I did not wish it, the limelight went unshared. So much credit must be given to George for everything he did for me, from caring for the children to bringing me milkshakes.

Being so near death and receiving the gift of faith so radically altered my perception of life that I came home from hospital a very different person from the woman he married.

On October 23, 1982, Nuria attended the Anthony Nolan Open Day with me. Supporters came from all over Britain to share in this event. A service in memory of Anthony was held in the chapel of St. Mary Abbot's Hospital. We came together to remember a brave little boy who suffered so much before he died but whose life has been used to save the lives of so many others. We came to honour the achievement of Shirley Nolan whose courage transformed her son's death into a monument of love and a symbol of hope. And we came to rejoice in three successful bone marrow transplants, all with unrelated donors who had been found through the Anthony Nolan Laboratories. For the six of us there were trophies, but it is impossible to say who really deserved them, the hard work and faithful prayers of so many were involved.

I accepted my trophy on behalf of all those who had made it possible for me to be there that day. I couldn't find words of my own to try to thank them. It was Jesus who spoke through my tears. 'Yesterday,' I told them, 'it was raining and I was out with my little three-year-old daughter. She was laughing with pure childish joy as she splashed in the puddles, and I was there to share in her delight. As you have done this for me, you have done it for the glory of my Father.'

I still have the GVH and I still go to the Westminster for regular check-ups. There I still sometimes see Mary or Donna or Valerie, but more often we see each other in our own homes. Jill is still with us, faithfully waiting on the Lord for her healing. Anna has become a born-again Christian. And Ian Kirby, my donor, continues to help with research into ITP.

On one of my check-ups I was introduced to a visiting Dutch doctor who was interested in my case. In describing the course of my illness, Dr. Joshi told him about the pneumonia and how it had completely disappeared 'by magic'.

'Dr. Joshi,' I said, 'you know it wasn't magic.' We smiled.

We both knew it was a miracle! It was a whole series of miracles on Horseferry Road that led to this complete victory over leukaemia. A miraculous achievement for all those involved medically. A victory for the prayers and faith of so many others.

But the greatest miracle of all was not my physical healing. This was *my* miracle – that God had given me a second chance to receive His love and His free gift of salvation, to receive His dear son Jesus into my life and heart.

*'And he will declare to his friends, 'I sinned, but God let me go. He did not let me die. I will go on living in the realm of light.'*

*'Yes, God often does these things for man – brings back his soul from the pit, so that he may live in the light of living.'*
*Job 33:27-30*

Oh, Lord, I praise You!

For assistance, further information, or donations:


Special Trustees of Westminster and Roehampton
Hospitals
Miriam Greenfell Fund
c/o Westminster Haematology Department
Westminster Hospital
London SW1
*Telephone*: 01-828 9811 ext 2012


Mrs Marian Matthews
The Anthony Nolan Laboratories
St Mary Abbots Hospital
Marloes Road
London W8 5LQ
*Telephone*: 01-937 2660


Leukaemia Research Fund
Dept. CW2
43 Great Ormond Street
London WC1N 3JJ
*Telephone*: 01-405 0101

*Other Marshall Pickering Paperbacks*

## THE TORN VEIL

*Sister Gulshan and Thelma Sangster*

Gulshan Fatima was brought up in a Muslim Sayed family according to the orthodox Islamic code of the Shias.

Suffering from a crippling paralysis she travelled to England in search of medical help. Although unsuccessful in medical terms, this trip marked the beginning of a spiritual awakening that led ultimately to her conversion to Christianity.

Gulshan and her father also travelled to Mecca in the hope that God would heal her, but that trip too was of no avail. However, Gulshan was not detered. She relentlessly pursued God and He faithfully answered her prayers. Her conversion, when it came, was dramatic and brought with a miraculous healing.

**The Torn Veil** is Sister Gulshan's thrilling testimony to the power of God which can break through every barrier.

# SURVIVOR

*Tania Kauppila*

Born into poverty, forced to endure filth and slave labour in a Nazi concentration camp, how did Tania Kauppila survive? When Nazi occupation forces arbitrarily decreed that one member from each family in the Russian city of Rovno must "serve the war effort" for a "three month" period in Germany, 12 year old Tania insisted that she be the one to go from her family. She was young and strong and her father was needed by her sick mother and younger brother.

At age 12, Tania had already experienced incredible hardships and had seen more of life's harsh realities than most women ever see. When she left her family – the only security she knew – she faced frightening, unanswerable questions. How would she survive? Would she ever see her family again? Would she ever find the God of her father? Would she ever find peace?

**Survivor** is the story of an incredible life spanning three continents and five decades. It is a witness to the sustaining strength and love of a God who will not let go.

If you wish to receive *regular*
*information* about *new books*,
please send your name and address
to:—
London Bible Warehouse
PO Box 123
Basingstoke
Hants RG23 7NL

Name: .....................................
Address: ...................................
...............................................
...............................................
...............................................

I am especially interested in:—

Music/Theology/"Popular"
Paperbacks
Delete which do not apply

P.S. If you have ideas for new Christian Books or
other products, Please write to us too!